Toxicity and Risk

Toxicity and Risk

Context, principles and practice

Paul Illing

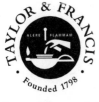

London and New York

First published 2001 by Taylor & Francis
11 New Fetter Lane, London EC4P 4EE

Simultaneously published in the USA and Canada
by Taylor & Francis Inc
29 West 35th Street, New York, NY 10001

Taylor & Francis is an imprint of the Taylor & Francis Group

© 2001 Paul Illing

Typeset in Sabon and Gill Sans by
Prepress Projects Ltd, Perth, Scotland
Printed and bound in Great Britain by
TJ International Ltd, Padstow, Cornwall

British Library Cataloguing in Publication Data
A catalogue record for this book is available from the British
Library

Library of Congress Cataloging in Publication Data
A catalog record has been requested

ISBN 0–415–23371–2

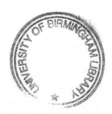

Contents

Preface

Like everything we touch, this book reflects experience. So, I had better state mine. The book reflects my experiences over some 30 years in toxic risk assessment, first in the pharmaceutical industry, more recently in a UK government regulatory agency and, most recently, as an academic and independent consultant.

The book has its origins in the late 1980s and early 1990s, when I first realised that there were two camps when it came to risk assessment. In the one camp, there were numerical risk assessors concerned with quantitative risk assessment. These seemed to me to be mainly engineers, but theirs was the 'accepted' view of how scientists were meant to think on risk matters. Then there was the view of the medical and toxicological communities, mainly judgemental and subjective but with – usually unstated – rules and procedures. The two did not mix at all easily, partly because the numerate and the literate often have difficulty talking to and understanding one another. They talk different languages. One aim of this book is to show that the concepts used in toxicological risk assessment can be expressed in both languages.

The second driver for developing ideas in this field was late one evening at a meeting of the British Toxicology Society. I had been well and truly chastised (by an administrator) for allowing society to overrule or not accept decisions by the technical experts. This encouraged me to look more closely at how toxicological risk assessment is managed, who does have the final say and how we go about decision-taking in order to benefit society. In this, the statement 'No (hu)man is an island' comes to mind, as does the idea that the freedom of individuals to do as they wish is trammelled by the need not to interfere with the rights of others. This is why the book paints a very broad picture, attempting to cover the context as well as the techniques of toxicological risk assessment.

The third reason was the obvious one: it seemed to me that there was a need for advanced students and practitioners (including myself) to have available a book that describes the principles and processes that they undertake when looking at the regulatory risk implications of their work.

The book may also be useful in trying to dispel the idea that toxicological risk assessment is a 'black art' by showing to non-practitioners that, however coarse the methods used, they do have an underlying basis of science and common sense. It could even start a debate on what we do, why and whether it is the most appropriate thing to do.

I owe much to mentors and colleagues over the years. I am indebted to my teachers, many years ago at Dundee University, for instilling their scepticism of 'given truth' and their ability to fierily debate honestly held minority opinions without rancour. I also thank the many colleagues over the years as they have (often unwittingly) passed ideas to me that have helped to form my view. However, the views expressed in this book are in no way their responsibility.

Finally, I thank the various authors and publishers who have granted permission for me to use their material, and the staff at Taylor & Francis who have gently kept me (nearly) up to scratch. The book would be the poorer without their help.

Paul Illing
June 2001

Acknowledgements

I am grateful to the following for permission to use their material:

New Scientist (Figure 2.2)
The Sunday Times (Figure 2.2)
Royal Society of Chemistry (Figure 2.10)
Copyright Unit, Her Majesty's Stationery Office (Figure 4.2)
Blackwell Publishers (Figure 5.2)
WHO Collaborating Centre for an International Clearing House for Major
Chemical Incidents (Figure 10.1)

Chapter 1

Introduction

Chemical substances are everywhere; they are present in the air that we breathe, in the food and water that we drink and eat and in the products that we make and consume. Chemical substances may be environmental (minerals, metal ores, atmospheric gases, natural products) or manufactured in origin. Some are safe to mine, manufacture or use, others are harmful. How does society and how do we decide what chemical substances to make, and when to use them? Also, the environment is full of chemical substances, some of which are harmful. How can control be exercised to prevent or minimise exposure to these chemicals? Taking decisions on how to manage exposure to toxic substances implies risk management, and, if risks are to be managed sensibly, risk assessment. The aim of this book is to set out the political, social, legal and scientific underpinning of risk assessment and risk management for toxic substances. Risk analysis is the field of study that covers this process, although it includes other areas of risk as well. Because the field is highly interdisciplinary, what is covered in the book and what is meant by the different terms used must be identified clearly.

What are toxicants (pollutants)?

Toxicology is the study of poisons. Toxicants (or pollutants) are agents which, when applied to a biological system, cause a deleterious perturbation to that system. In other words, there is a harmful interaction between an agent and a biological system. The agent may be chemical, physical or biological in origin. It may be studied to ensure toxicity is manifest in the intended circumstances or to ensure safety (Figure 1.1). Although the principles of risk management apply to all forms of agent, this book will concentrate on agents involving a chemical interaction, i.e. chemical substances, including many of natural origin. The organisational level at which the interaction is investigated can range from the molecule to the biosphere (Figure 1.2), with human ill-health and environmental degradation being the outcomes of the interaction.

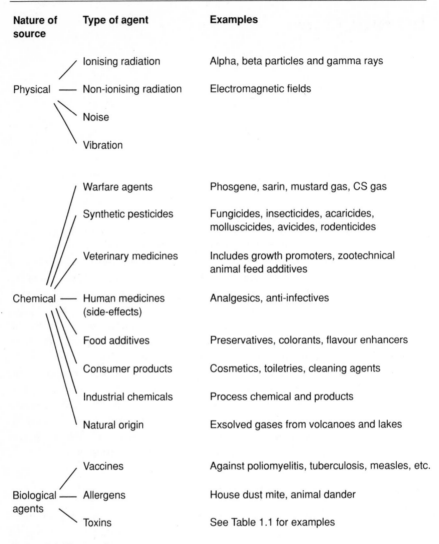

Nature of source	Type of agent	Examples
Physical	Ionising radiation	Alpha, beta particles and gamma rays
	Non-ionising radiation	Electromagnetic fields
	Noise	
	Vibration	
Chemical	Warfare agents	Phosgene, sarin, mustard gas, CS gas
	Synthetic pesticides	Fungicides, insecticides, acaricides, molluscicides, avicides, rodenticides
	Veterinary medicines	Includes growth promoters, zootechnical animal feed additives
	Human medicines (side-effects)	Analgesics, anti-infectives
	Food additives	Preservatives, colorants, flavour enhancers
	Consumer products	Cosmetics, toiletries, cleaning agents
	Industrial chemicals	Process chemical and products
	Natural origin	Exsolved gases from volcanoes and lakes
Biological agents	Vaccines	Against poliomyelitis, tuberculosis, measles, etc.
	Allergens	House dust mite, animal dander
	Toxins	See Table 1.1 for examples

Figure 1.1 Types of toxic agents.

Chemical agents include many natural substances as well as industrially produced synthetic chemicals and their degradation products. Some very poisonous substances are of natural origin – these include bacterial and fungal toxins, toxins of plant origin, spider poisons, snake venoms and poisons derived from fish (Table 1.1). Other poisons are derived from the chemical laboratory. They include substances intended to be poisonous to pests or disease-causing organisms, as well as chemicals which are intended for other uses and which happen also to be hazardous. Synthetic chemicals

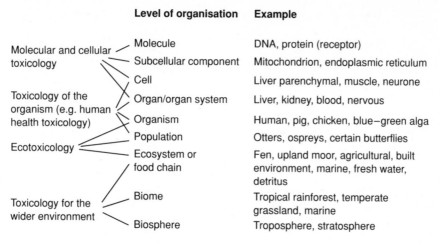

Level of organisation	Example

Molecular and cellular toxicology

Toxicology of the organism (e.g. human health toxicology)

Ecotoxicology

Toxicology for the wider environment

Molecule — DNA, protein (receptor)

Subcellular component — Mitochondrion, endoplasmic reticulum

Cell — Liver parenchymal, muscle, neurone

Organ/organ system — Liver, kidney, blood, nervous

Organism — Human, pig, chicken, blue–green alga

Population — Otters, ospreys, certain butterflies

Ecosystem or food chain — Fen, upland moor, agricultural, built environment, marine, fresh water, detritus

Biome — Tropical rainforest, temperate grassland, marine

Biosphere — Troposphere, stratosphere

Figure 1.2 Levels of biological organisation. The first column gives a description of the type of toxicology being undertaken when examining the particular level of organisation, although it should be noted that there is considerable overlap.

are produced in and may be consumed by chemical processes, thus process safety must be considered alongside product safety.

The interaction between a substance and a biological system can be beneficial, neutral or harmful. Beneficial interactions are the aim when eating and drinking or when taking chemicals (drugs) to cure illness. Ideally, these interactions result in the maintenance or restoration of homeostasis in the organism. Harmful interactions (to the organism or system being targeted, or to the organism affected incidentally or affected accidentally by the chemical) are those which result in loss of homeostasis, leading to debility, damage or death. That harmful interaction may be with humans, with other species or with the wider environment. The interaction may be studied at many levels, from molecular interactions to interactions affecting the overall ability of earth to support present-day life (Figure 1.2). The undesirable effects caused by these interactions are the toxic hazards associated with the chemicals. The types of evidence of toxicity used for risk assessment, and the way in which the evidence is taken into a risk assessment, will be examined in Chapters 7, 8 and 10–12.

Harm, hazard and risk

Harm, hazard and risk are important concepts in risk analysis. They have been defined by many bodies, and an international committee – the Interagency Organisation for the Management of Chemicals (a joint body supported by the Organisation of Economic Co-operation and Development and the United Nations International Programme on Chemical Safety) – is

Table 1.1 Examples of toxins and venoms (toxic substances from biological
sources)

Source	Species	Toxin
Higher plants	Castor oil plant (*Ricinus communis*)	Ricin
	Deadly nightshade (*Atropa belladonna*)	Belladonna alkaloids (atropine)
Fungi	e.g. *Aspergillus* spp.	Mycotoxins (aflatoxins in peanuts, tricothecanes) – food contaminants/ potential warfare agents
Blue–green algae (cyanobacteria)	*Anabena, Microcystis, Nostoc, Oscillatoria* spp., etc.	Toxins produced by algal blooms in nutrient-rich water under axenic growth conditions, e.g. microcystins (hepatotoxins)
Bacteria	*Clostridium botulinus*	Botulinum toxin ('lockjaw')
	Escherichia coli (O157)	Verotoxin (nephrotoxin) (food poisoning due to contamination with organisms producing the toxins)
Molluscs (shellfish)	*Gonyalux* spp. and *Pyridinium* spp. (dinoflagellates)	Saxitoxin produced by dinoflagellates in contaminated bivalve molluscs (oyster, clam, mussel) causing paralytic shellfish poisoning
Arthropods (arachnids – spiders)	*Lactrodectus mactans* (black widow)	Neurotoxic venom
Reptiles (snakes)	Coral snakes, cobras, mambas, kraits, sea snakes (*Elapidae*)	Neurotoxic venom
Fish	Puffer fish	Tetrodotoxin (ingestion results in neurotransmission block)
	Stingrays, weever fish	Venom from spines on fins causes intense, incapacitating pain following sting

Sources: Ballantyne *et al.* (1999), Bell and Codd (1996), Chan (1997).

attempting to set up an internationally acceptable set of definitions. A series
of definitions is given in Table 1.2. Perhaps the best way of combining the
definitions is: '*risk* is the possibility of suffering *harm* from a *hazard*'. The
most general definitions of risk include insurance risks, economic risks, risks

from geological events and bad weather, and wider engineering risks (e.g. aircraft safety) as well as risks arising from substances, whether manufactured or of natural origin.

As can be seen from Table 1.2, hazard is an intrinsic property of a process, situation or substance. Potential chemical hazards include the ability to cause fires and explosions, and to corrode pipework and tanks in chemical plant, as well as to cause ill-health and environmental degradation. This book is concerned solely with toxicity (ill-health and environmental degradation), thus these other hazards will not be considered further. Furthermore, the level of effect seen for a toxic hazard depends on the amount of the chemical (dose) to which the biological system is exposed. Hence, it is necessary to consider how much of the chemical is needed to cause a particular level of

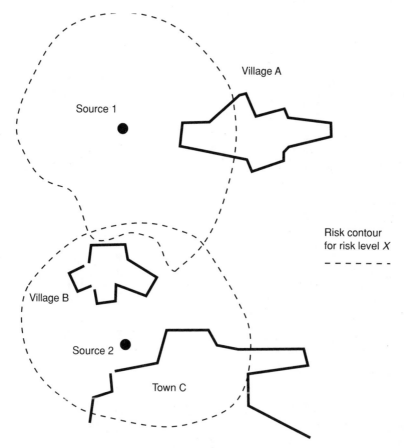

Figure 1.3   The difference between individual risk and societal risk. Although the same individual risk level (to humans) will exist for sources 1 and 2, the greater population around source 2 owing to the presence of town C will result in higher levels of societal risk.

Table 1.2 Definitions of hazard, harm and risk

Source	Hazard	Risk	Reference/ additional information
OECD/IPCS project on harmonisation of hazard/risk assessment terminology	Inherent property of an agent or situation capable of having adverse effects on something. Hence, the substance, agent, source of energy or situation having that property	The probability of adverse effects caused under specified circumstances by an agent in an organism, a population or an ecological system	Lewalle (1999)
US Presidential/ Congressional Commission on Risk Assessment and Management	A source of possible damage or injury	The probability of a specific outcome, generally adverse, given a particular set of conditions	US Presidential/ Congressional Commission on Risk Assessment Management (1997)
International Union of Pure and Applied Chemistry (IUPAC) Commission on Toxicology	Set of inherent properties of a substance, mixture of substances or a process involving substances that, underproduction, usage or disposal conditions, make it capable of causing adverse effects to organisms or the environment, depending on the degree of exposure	1 Possibility that a harmful effect (death, injury or loss) arising from exposure to a chemical or physical agent may occur under specific conditions 2 Expected frequency of occurrence of a harmful event (death, injury or loss) arising from exposure to a chemical or physical agent under specific conditions	Duffus (1993)

Royal Society	The situation that in particular circumstances could lead to harm, where harm is the loss to a human being, etc. consequent on damage and damage is the loss of inherent quality suffered by an entity (physical or biological)	A combination of the frequency of occurrence of a defined hazard and the magnitude of the consequences of that occurrence	Royal Society Study Group (1992)
Institution of Chemical Engineers	A physical situation with a potential for human injury, damage to property, damage to the environment or some combination of these	The likelihood of a specified undesired event within a specified period or in specified circumstances. It may be either a *frequency* (the number of specified events occurring in unit time) or a *probability* (the probability of a specified event following a prior event), depending on circumstances	Jones (1992)

harm, and this leads to dose–effect and dose–response relationships and the need to consider exposure when examining risk. The ways in which exposure is included in risk assessment are considered in Chapters 9–12. Often, exposure and toxicity are intimately linked, and are considered in the same chapter.

In practice, two further distinctions are useful. These are 'individual risk' and 'societal risk' or 'population risk'. Individual risk is the risk to the individual, and is a simple statement of probability of an event occurring, wherever placed. Societal or population risk is the risk associated with size (e.g. numbers killed) as well as frequency of event. Societal risk is concerned with events which exceed a certain size, and hence come to public awareness because of their severity; population risk is when events may result in danger of loss of all or a large part of a population of a species. Both are therefore tied to population 'at risk' and hence population densities in geographic areas. The difference between individual and societal (population) risk is illustrated in Figure 1.3.

For many purposes, such as human health and the licensing of products and standard setting, or when dealing with small numbers of an endangered species, it is possible to deal in terms of individual risk. For other purposes,

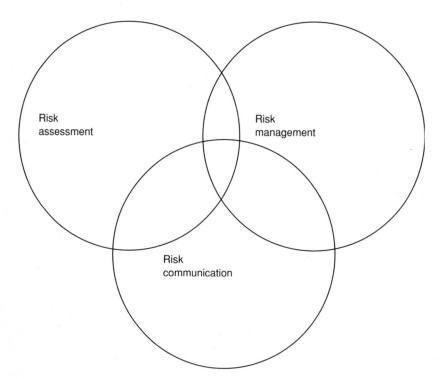

Figure 1.4 Relationships among risk assessment, risk management and risk communication.

numbers of individuals, and hence societal (or population) risk, become important. This is especially true when dealing with the potential for human ill-health following major accidents and with effects on individual species, food webs and ecosystems in the environment.

Risk assessment, risk management and risk communication

There are three major elements in any attempt to manage risks. These are risk assessment, risk management and risk communication (Figure 1.4). All three are iterative and interactive, i.e. they depend on one another and when one changes the others need to be re-examined to ensure that they are still suitable. A term that can be used to describe this process is risk analysis (Lewalle, 1999).

Risk analysis is not carried out within a vacuum. There are philosophical and political processes underlying risk assessment and risk management, which involve decisions by society concerning the rights and duties of individuals and organisations. When the risks are associated with the use of chemicals, society – through a political and legislative process – may take a

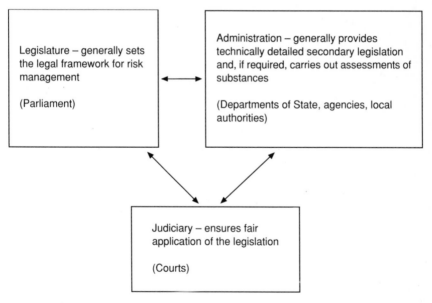

Figure 1.5 Relationships among the different arms of government. The examples of the organs of government carrying out these functions are those for the UK; in the USA, the distinction between legislature and administration is much clearer because, although the political heads of government departments in the UK are members of the majority party in Parliament, in the USA they are not members of the legislature.

judgement concerning the balance of rights and duties between individuals and organisations, or it may decide that, in the interests of good government, the administrative arm of government should undertake the risk management on behalf of society as a whole. How that administrative arm approaches the risk management depends on the philosophy (or philosophies) within which the regulatory approach is framed. The judicial system is used to ensure that society (and the administrators) adheres to the requirements placed upon it through law. The interactions of these arms of government are shown in Figure 1.5. The processes are examined in Chapters 2–6.

Part I

The context in which toxic risk analysis takes place

Chapter 2

What risk management covers

Risk management covers a very wide sphere of activities. Risk management has been defined as 'the making of decisions concerning risk and their subsequent implementation' (Royal Society Study Group, 1983). The US Presidential/Congressional Commission on Risk Assessment and Risk Management (1997: vol. 1) gave a more exhaustive definition:

> **Risk management** is the process of identifying, evaluating, selecting and implementing actions to reduce risks to human health and ecosystems. The goal of risk management is scientifically sound, cost effective, integrated actions that reduce or prevent risks while taking into account social, cultural, ethical, political and legal considerations.

And the Organisation for Economic Co-operation and Development (OECD)/International Programme on Chemical Safety (IPCS) project on the harmonisation of hazard/risk terminology states (Lewalle, 1999):

> Risk management: Decision making process involving considerations of political, social, economic and technical factors with relevant risk assessment information relating to hazard so as to develop, analyse and compare regulatory and non-regulatory options and select and implement the optimal response for safety from that hazard.

This third definition explicitly recognises that political, social and economic factors, as well as technical factors, affect how risks are managed. Risk includes economic risks, insurance risks, engineering risks, risk from natural events and risk from industrial activities, so risk management is a term that can be used to describe how any of these activities are handled. Here, we are concerned with agent-induced health risks and risks to the environment. The aims of this type of health risk management are:

- to protect health, preferably by preventing ill-health due to physical, chemical or biological agents, but also by providing protective measures and appropriate treatments in the event of ill-health occurring;

- to deal with public health concerns over the toxic potential of particular agents and processes.

Risk management for effects on the environment can be similarly described as being:

- to protect the environment, preferably by preventing environmental pollution, but also by providing suitable protective measures to prevent damage arising from pollution, and appropriate remediation procedures to repair damage, once caused;
- to deal with public concerns over potential causes of environmental pollution.

Health and environmental risks may be those due to accidental or anticipatable exposure to hazardous chemicals (Figure 2.1). Accidental risks can be divided into risks where small-scale loss of control may occur or risks where there is potential for a major incident. Anticipatable risks include those arising from deliberate exposure to a chemical, usually for a specific reason, as well as those arising incidentally, either directly or indirectly.

Before risks can be managed, they have to be assessed. Knowledge of both the likely hazard and probable levels of exposure are required in order to assess these risks. Health risks can be divided into occupational and public health risks. Both types of risk can occur when dealing with process safety. In addition, public health includes the human health aspects of product safety and environmental pollution. Essentially, these are all areas where knowledge of hazard is provided by various specialists in human health, including, notably, toxicologists. Environmental risk includes pollution principally affecting ecosystems and non-human species as well as atmospheric pollution, and hence includes knowledge of hazards obtained by ecotoxicologists and environmental chemists. Risk management therefore includes managing risks following a risk evaluation. This sort of risk is called *objective* (or statistical) *risk*.

In many circumstances, it is necessary to manage perceived risk as well as objective risk. *Perceived risk* can be considered as that risk thought by an individual or group to be present in a given situation (Jones, 1992). Risk perception involves both feelings and judgements, but it need not include an objective risk assessment. Figure 2.2 illustrates the headlines that ensue when 'perceived' risk and 'objective' risk differ. Risk communication needs to be managed just as effectively as risk assessment if society is to organise itself using decisions based on evidence, rather than on instinct. This aspect of risk management will be addressed more thoroughly in Chapter 5.

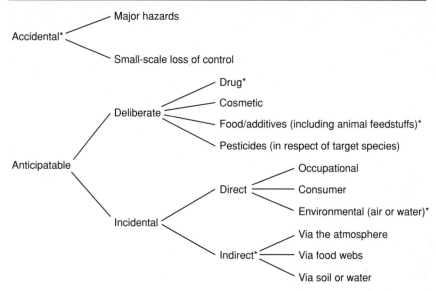

Figure 2.1   A classification of potential exposures to chemicals. *These exposure routes are relevant to other species as well as humans. From Koundakjian and Illing (1992), with amendments.

National and international bodies

Risk management has to cover both the management of objective/statistical risks and the management of perceived risks. Thus, within governments and international organisations, it includes:

- developing policies on how to handle different types of risk;
- management of agent-induced health or environmental pollution-based risk issues, whether they are based on objective or on perceived risk assessments;
- regulation of individual risks.

Within policies for handling different risks will be a policy on how to communicate on risk issues. Once upon a time, *ex cathedra* statements from government or scientists were sufficient, but they have become unacceptable in recent years (see Figure 2.2). Much more emphasis has to be placed on communication as a multidirectional transfer of information in order to ensure convergence between the 'official' view and the public perception of the risk and how it should be managed. This is discussed further in Chapter 5.

Risk management includes decisions concerning the need for regulatory schemes and the type of scheme that should be implemented. Many schemes

THE SUNDAY TIMES

More weasel words

Will Whitehall never learn? The health department's bland assurance that the risk to children vaccinated with a suspect polio vaccine of catching the human variant of mad cow disease is "incalculably small" shows it has not learnt. We have been fobbed off with this sort of phrase before. It is Whitehall-speak for: "Well, yes, there may be some risk but it's so small we can't actually measure it and, even if we could (or have), there's no need for alarm. Take our word for it."

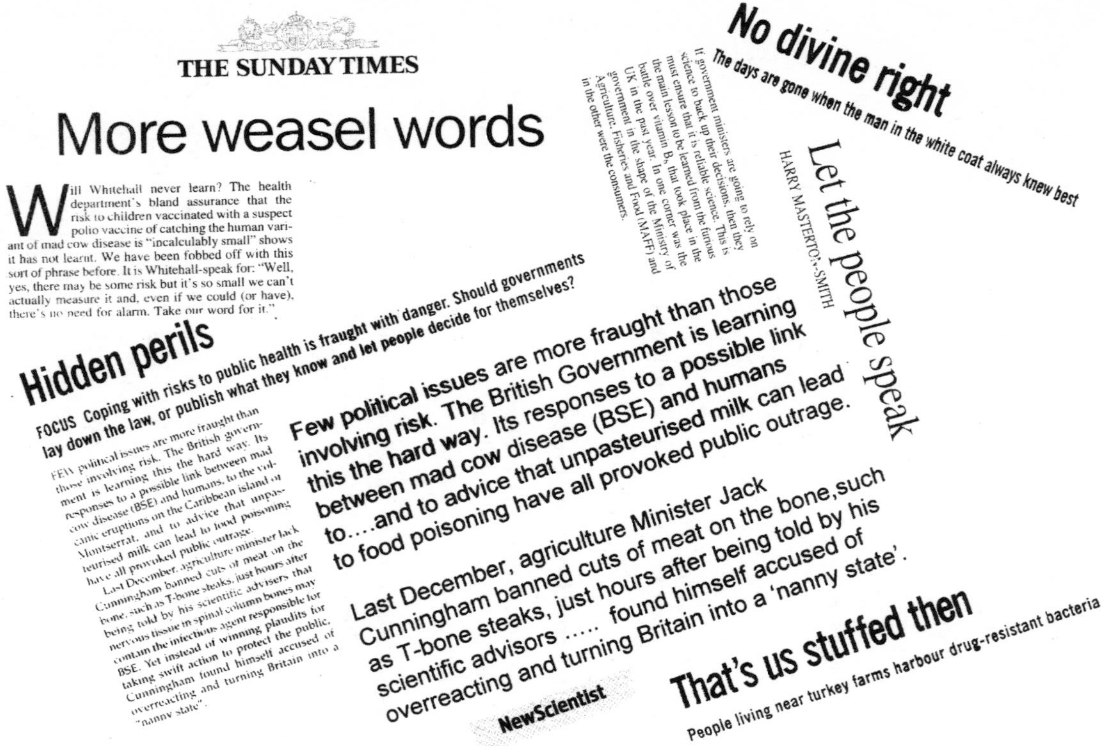

No divine right

The days are gone when the man in the white coat always knew best

If government ministers are going to rely on science to back up their decisions, then they must ensure that it is reliable science. This is the main lesson to be learned from the furious battle over vitamin B_6 that took place in the UK in the past year. In one corner was the government in the shape of the Ministry of Agriculture, Fisheries and Food (MAFF) and in the other were the consumers.

Let the people speak

HARRY MASTERTON-SMITH

Hidden perils

FOCUS Coping with risks to public health is fraught with danger. Should governments lay down the law, or publish what they know and let people decide for themselves?

FEW political issues are more fraught than those involving risk. The British government is learning this the hard way. Its responses to a possible link between mad cow disease (BSE) and humans, to the volcanic eruptions on the Caribbean island of Montserrat, and to advice that unpasteurised milk can lead to food poisoning have all provoked public outrage.

Last December, agriculture minister Jack Cunningham banned cuts of meat on the bone, such as T-bone steaks, just hours after being told by his scientific advisers that nervous tissue in spinal column bones may contain the infectious agent responsible for BSE. Yet instead of winning plaudits for taking swift action to protect the public, Cunningham found himself accused of overreacting and turning Britain into a "nanny state".

Few political issues are more fraught than those involving risk. The British Government is learning this the hard way. Its responses to a possible link between mad cow disease (BSE) and humans to....and to advice that unpasteurised milk can lead to food poisoning have all provoked public outrage.

Last December, agriculture Minister Jack Cunningham banned cuts of meat on the bone, such as T-bone steaks, just hours after being told by his scientific advisors ..... found himself accused of overreacting and turning Britain into a 'nanny state'.

NewScientist

That's us stuffed then

People living near turkey farms harbour drug-resistant bacteria

Figure 2.2 Newspaper and magazine headlines on health risks. The headlines are concerned with the difference between 'objective' and 'perceived' risk and the consequent lack of acceptability of the proposed risk-management procedure. Issues include poliomyelitis vaccine, vitamin B_6, antibiotics in animal feedstuffs, unpasteurised milk, 'mad cow' disease [bovine spongiform encephalitis (BSE)/variant Creutzfeldt-Jakob disease] and the general principle that scientists are not always right. The headlines include claimed overreaction (vitamin B_6, BSE and T-bone steaks) as well as underreaction. From the *New Scientist* and *The Sunday Times*.

involve 'permissioning', agreeing to employ an industrial process, accepting a 'safety case' or deciding on the acceptability of a particular land use (Box 2.1). It can also be for use of an agent or for a substance to be present in a product, in the food chain or in the wider environment following acceptance of a notification, granting of a licence or placing on an approved list. It includes setting standards for additives and contaminants. It also includes standard setting in the absence of permission, as with standard setting for public and occupational health and environmental pollution purposes (Box 2.2). These standards may be set for different parts of the chain from source, through the pathway by which the chemical is transmitted to the receptor.

Box 2.1 'Permissioning' systems involving potential toxicants or environmental pollutants.

Product safety	
Licensing	Human medicines
	Veterinary products
	Plant protection products
	Biocides
Placing on an approved list	Food additives
	Cosmetics ingredients
Notification	New chemicals
	High production volume 'existing' chemicals
Process safety	Integrated pollution prevention and control
Land use (including planning)	Waste disposal
	Reuse of contaminated land
	Major industrial hazards
	Developments around major industrial hazards

Box 2.2 Standards derived from standard setting.

'Input' standards	Maximum residue levels (MRL; foods)
	Discharge limits (air, water)
'Intake' standards	Acceptable daily intake (ADI; food additives)
	Tolerable daily intake (TDI; food and drinking water contaminants)
	Environmental quality standards (air, water, soil)
	Indoor air quality
	Occupational exposure standard (workplace)
	Maximum exposure limit (workplace)
'Uptake' standards	Biological exposure index/health guidance value (workplace; e.g. blood lead level)

Note
'Permissioning' may be accompanied by concomitant standard setting, and standards may be set for agents not subject to 'permissioning'.

Standards for emission from the source can be described as 'input' standards; standards based on measurements on the ambient medium (air breathed, water drunk, food eaten, i.e. the pathway) as 'intake' standards; and standards based on the concentrations in the organism (measured in urine, in exhaled air, in blood, etc. as the nearest that can be achieved to measurement at the receptor within the organism) as 'uptake' standards. The appropriate standard is dependent on the stage at which control is being exercised (Figure 2.3).

Often, risk management is aimed at controlling specific processes or products in clearly specified circumstances (pollution hazards, drugs, pesticides). The approach used by regulatory authorities for many toxic

Source	Input	Pathway	Intake	Uptake	Receptor
Point	Emission limit	Environment	Exposure limit (outdoor, indoor air, drinking water, occupational)		Biosphere (biodiversity)
	Discharge limit	Environmental medium (air, water, soil)/ ecosystem		Biological exposure index	Species
Diffuse	Maximum residue level/limit (for individual food or site)	Food basket (total diet) and drinking water	Daily/weekly/ annual intake		Organism (e.g. humans)

Figure 2.3   The passage of a chemical from source to receptor and the standards that can be used when controlling exposure to that chemical. Notes: (1) The input from a source may be accidental or anticipated (see Chapter 2). For accidental releases, the emphasis is on the identification of the size and duration of the potential release in order to determine the ways in which the likely end-effects can be minimised and prevented. For anticipated releases, the emphasis is to identify the likely end-effects in order to determine the acceptable (or tolerable) pattern for releases. (2) 'Pathway' may include the dispersion pattern, transfer between environmental media, bioconcentration, etc. that may occur between the emission of the chemical from a source and the take up by the receptor. For food safety, 'pathway' is the way in which different individual foods (and their containments) are aggregated to obtain the total food intake. (3) In the case of a biosphere, the source (e.g. greenhouse gases, chlorofluorocarbons) is diffuse, mixing occurs in the atmosphere and control is exercised at source through international agreements concerning the production of the pollutant. (4) For an ecosystem, input and intake are, in effect, the same. For individual species within the ecosystem, a model for the ecosystem contains the pathways by which the pollutant moves through the ecosystem, the effects that the pollutant has on the individual species present, and hence the effect that it has on the balance and diversity of species present.

risks can be described as preventative – ensuring, as far as possible, protection in order to avoid, so far as is practicable, the likelihood of a substance or process being allowed for use when in fact it is not safe to do so. Frequently, standard setting has been conducted piecemeal, but more holistic approaches to risk management are now being considered. These include 'life cycle analysis' (process or product), 'integrated pollution prevention and control' (IPPC) for industrial processes and 'integrated pest and pesticide management' (IPPM) for plant protection products. Even with the best risk-management procedures there will be residual risks, such as those from accidents or those not evaluated because they have not been identified.

Similar risk-management issues will affect large, multinational companies. There will need to be common approaches across the whole company, and often beyond, to risk issues and standards. Companies often use generic approaches using titles such as 'responsible care' or 'product stewardship' to emphasise their commitment to dealing properly with risk management.

Local government and individual companies/sites

Agenda 21 is the drive for a better world originating from the United Nations Conference on Environmental Development (Rio; the 'Earth Summit'). Local Authorities are involved in risk management involving toxic risks. They are particularly involved in attempts to achieve 'sustainable development' through: reducing waste and promoting recycling; saving energy and conserving water; cutting down on noise and pollution; planning urban regeneration; and developing and maintaining biodiversity. National government sets the toxic risk assessment and policy; local authorities develop the detailed plans for their local areas and implement their local plans. Similar planning is often undertaken by industrial companies in order to fulfil their role in implementing this agenda.

Chapter 3

Legal and organisational frameworks

Most risk management, and hence risk assessment, takes place within a legal context, a set of rules designed for the good of those living within a particular society. The legal context takes, as its starting point, the State, and varies from State to State, although recent developments internationally mean that much of that context has become internationalised.

There are two parts to any legal system, statute law and some form of basic law, such as the common law (for England and Wales and the USA), Roman law (Scotland and, through Code Napoléon, most of Europe) or the sharia (in many Muslim countries). This may be supplemented by international law on human rights. Generally, statute law is the law created by the legislature – the law-making body; the legal framework that underlies governmental risk assessment and risk management is based on statute law.

In the UK, statute law includes a mixture of international treaties and conventions, European Union directives and regulations, and UK acts of Parliament and regulations. The laws concerned with the basic rights of individuals (in common law, the torts of nuisance and negligence) are the basis of litigation concerned with interference in the use and enjoyment of another's land or injury to health through exposure to harmful agents.

Statute law

How legislation is enacted depends on the national system of government. Often, legislation is a response to a perceived need, frequently a need identified as a consequence of a disaster. In most systems, there is primary legislation, setting out the principles of what should be covered and the penalties for failure to comply, and secondary legislation, containing greater detail on what needs to be undertaken in order to comply with the primary legislation.

UK law

The primary legislation in the UK takes the form of acts of Parliament.

These set up regulatory systems and, usually, give a framework under which subsidiary legislation (regulations, etc.) can be drafted and enacted. Members of Parliament (or, indeed, of any legislature) are elected by the public to represent their interests. Thus, the legislature is a mechanism to ensure that, overall, the public interest is served by any statute-based regulatory system.

Generally, legislation is developed to deal with a perceived need. Legislation to control medicines was one consequence of several very public cases of medicines having unacceptable side-effects. Health and safety legislation has often been the consequence of disaster – examples include Flixborough (Health and Safety at Work, etc. Act 1974), Seveso (European Directives on Major Hazards) and Piper alpha (legislation concerning the offshore oil industry). The legislation introducing the Food Standards Agency was the consequence of disquiet concerning food safety, fuelled by public discussion of a number of incidents (an *Escherichia coli* O157 food poisoning episode in Lanarkshire, 'mad cow disease'), and issues (disquiet concerning food additives and contaminants and labelling). The process of developing UK legislation is given in Figure 3.1.

Parliament debates acts of Parliament; regulations are 'laid' before Parliament by being placed in the library. These are only debated if Parliament calls for it, and, in the absence of debate, come into force about 30 days after being laid. This division of labour is inevitable as Members of Parliament (or, indeed, any legislature) are generalists elected by the public to represent the interests, and regulations often contain material requiring detailed specialist knowledge.

When dealing with toxicological risk assessment, there will also be guidance on how to comply with the regulations and on what information is required under the regulations. Although not available generally, in the health and safety field subordinate 'approved codes of practice' (which can have a special place in law) are also possible. Approval is by the Health and Safety Commission, i.e. one further step removed from the legislature. Neither guidance nor approved codes of practice are placed before Parliament. An example of this multilayered approach is given in Table 3.1.

Often, different pieces of legislation are required for different parts of the UK. Normally, legislation is passed separately for Northern Ireland, and sometimes the legislation has to be written in such a way that it is applicable in the different circumstances pertaining under Scots law, with its different structures and processes. With the coming of delegated powers to Scotland and Wales, the detailed supervision of the operation of much of the legislation has been handed over to these devolved assemblies.

European Union and international law

National legislation is not the only source of law. Often, legislation has been passed ceding authority in toxicological risk assessment and

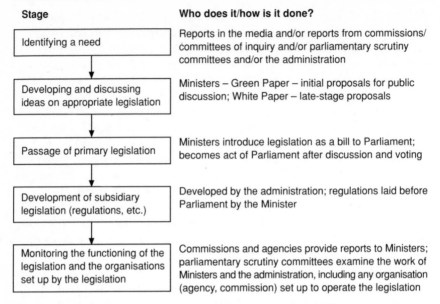

Stage	Who does it/how is it done?
Identifying a need	Reports in the media and/or reports from commissions/committees of inquiry and/or parliamentary scrutiny committees and/or the administration
Developing and discussing ideas on appropriate legislation	Ministers – Green Paper – initial proposals for public discussion; White Paper – late-stage proposals
Passage of primary legislation	Ministers introduce legislation as a bill to Parliament; becomes act of Parliament after discussion and voting
Development of subsidiary legislation (regulations, etc.)	Developed by the administration; regulations laid before Parliament by the Minister
Monitoring the functioning of the legislation and the organisations set up by the legislation	Commissions and agencies provide reports to Ministers; parliamentary scrutiny committees examine the work of Ministers and the administration, including any organisation (agency, commission) set up to operate the legislation

Figure 3.1 Development and monitoring of legislation in the UK.

management to regional bodies, such as the European Union (EU), or to international bodies, such as the United Nations, the World Trade Organisation and OECD.

Generally, there is an underlying treaty or convention negotiated by the national administrations which is then passed through national legislatures and, if required, wider regional legislative assemblies. For example, the underlying treaties setting up and modifying the EU (Rome, Maastricht, Nice, etc.) are negotiated by the administrations of each State and have to be agreed by the legislatures of all the States participating in the EU. In some cases, the general public also has to confirm the decision to accept treaty provisions through a referendum.

The treaties allow the EU Council (of ministers of the individual States), the European Parliament and the European Commission rights to create subordinate legislation (directives and EU regulations). There are three areas within the treaties that have resulted in legislation involving toxicological risk assessment. These are:

1   Establishing the single market – maintaining the free market in goods and services; differences in classification and labelling requirements for health and environmental risks would constitute non-tariff barriers to trade; as standards set are intended to be high standards, individual States cannot set tougher standards.
2   Action on the health and safety of workers – setting minimum standards for health and safety throughout the EU; States must meet these minimum standards, they can set tougher standards if they so wish.

Table 3.1 An example of the different levels of UK legislative instrument

Type of document	Example	Comment
Act of Parliament	Health and Safety at Work, etc. Act 1974	
	European Community Act 1972	This act allows EU directives to be entered into UK regulations without having to introduce new acts of Parliament when directives are wider than the areas covered by the parent act under which the regulations are made
Regulations	Chemicals (Hazard Information and Packaging) Regulations, 1994 Notification of New Substances Regulations, 1993	
Approved codes of practice	Safety data sheets for substances and preparations dangerous for supply (Health and Safety Commission, 1994)	The Health and Safety at Work, etc. Act 1974 gives a special place in law to approved codes of practice: if someone has not followed the relevant provisions of an approved code of practice, they have to show that they have complied with the law in some other way in order to demonstrate that they are not in breach of health and safety law
Guidance on regulations		Approved guide to the classification and labelling of substances and preparations dangerous for supply (Health and Safety Commission, 1999)

Note
General principles for legislation on health and safety and the environment can be obtained from the introductory sections of the most recent edition of appropriate legal texts such as Duxbury and Morton (2000), Hendy and Ford (1998) and Hughes (1996).

3   Action on the environment to preserve, protect and improve it and to contribute towards protecting human health – setting high standards.

Although EU regulations override the laws of individual States, directives have to be incorporated into the legislation of the individual States. Directives come in two forms – council directives, setting frameworks, and commission directives, filling in the detail. The legislatures for each State have to create a means by which EU directives can be translated into the individual State's law. The European Communities Act of 1972 is the underlying act used to translate directives into UK law when no more specific legislation is available. Generally, UK regulations, with or without advisory codes of practice, are the device by which the directives are translated into UK law.

Non-EU sources of international law can be divided into 'hard law' and 'soft law'. Treaty provisions give rise to 'hard law'. International organisations may also have powers under a treaty to bind the parties to the treaty by their decisions. Examples include:

1   the International Maritime Organisation (transport of hazardous substances);
2   the Oslo and Paris Commissions countering pollution threats to the North Sea and the north-eastern Atlantic;
3   the World Trade Organisation in respect of trade of foodstuffs and hence acceptable levels of food additives and contaminants in foods traded internationally.

Recommendations or declarations made by international conferences or intergovernmental organisations are 'soft law'. 'Soft laws' fix norms of behaviour but are not binding in the same way as 'hard law'.

Differences from the USA

In the USA, the primary split is between the individual State and the Union as a whole. The US Congress acts to provide reserve provisions, but a State retains the right, for example, to set its own occupational health and environmental standards. The US Congress passes acts, and the appropriate US Wide Agency produces regulations. However, there is a crucial difference between European practice and that in the USA. Technically, the legislature and the administration are separated in both systems. However, in Europe, where the Prime Minister/ministers are drawn from the majority political party or coalition of parties, difficulties and loopholes in legislation can be plugged rapidly by the governing ministers who can introduce legislation and drive it through with their majority in the legislature. This is not possible in the USA. The US Executive (President and Secretaries of Departments) is rigidly separated from the legislature (Congress) and cross-membership is minimal. The legislature first has to be convinced by the Executive (not the same people and often from a different political grouping) that legislation is needed. Thus, challenging legislation in the courts is more useful in the USA as, should the court decision highlight a loophole, the speed with which it can be plugged is so much slower.

As a consequence of the rigid separation of legislature and executive, there has been a 'technicalising' of toxicological risk assessment in the USA, with technical rules and rigidities being developed to overcome the difficulties posed by societal concerns and legislative loopholes. This technical approach has been further encouraged by Congress's use of committees of the National Research Council to investigate risk assessment and management for toxicological risks, and the reports derived from these committees (for some examples of reports, see National Research Council, 1983, 1994, 1996). European toxicological risk assessment remains more flexible. There is less need to use purely technical, rule-based approaches to decision-taking for mixed technical and societal decisions in order to render them defensible in court. Although hitherto it has been possible to maintain greater flexibility and to use more pragmatism when handling 'technical judgements', and hence to allow for political or societal inputs to be taken more readily into the system, the need for consistency within the European system is reducing this flexibility.

Management systems

Regulatory management of toxic agents is rarely simple, and systems usually cross government departmental boundaries. Essentially, there is a matrical system of regulation. Most governments have their own regulatory system that feeds into the international standards setting. In the UK, there is a series of committees involved in the regulatory management system (Figure 3.2). These committees advise ministers who undertake (or delegate to officials who then undertake on the minister's behalf) the executive action. The committees can be divided into two groups. The first group comprises those committees concerned with providing a more directed input into policy than is possible through Parliament about societal and ethical concerns on issues in particular fields, and on how to handle them. The second group of committees is responsible for recommending specific actions following detailed assessments of, frequently, individual substances intended for named purposes. These committees consist of independent experts in their field (usually academics) and representatives of various bodies affected by the decisions ('stakeholders'), and are supported by secretariats that include appropriate technical expertise. If the personnel chosen to be members of these committees are opinion leaders in their fields, their conclusions will be representative of the relevant scientific, technical and societal opinion. Often, the actual committee sets up subcommittees and working parties to deal with specific aspects of the business of the committee. Committees may delegate authority to the secretariat to decide the simplest cases on the basis of agreed guidelines. These national committees also feed into the now internationalised standard setting by regional and international bodies (Box 3.1). Within each of these levels, there is a matrix of agreements, advice and guidance aimed at providing the framework for conducting the risk management.

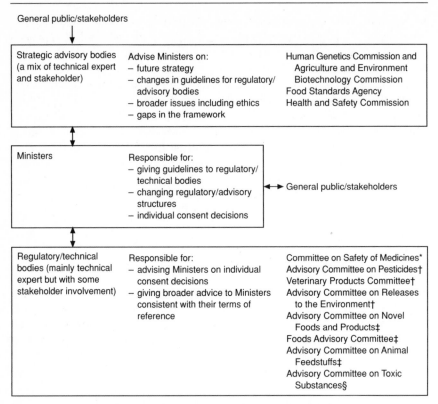

General public/stakeholders

| Strategic advisory bodies (a mix of technical expert and stakeholder) | Advise Ministers on:
– future strategy
– changes in guidelines for regulatory/ advisory bodies
– broader issues including ethics
– gaps in the framework | Human Genetics Commission and Agriculture and Environment Biotechnology Commission
Food Standards Agency
Health and Safety Commission |

| Ministers | Responsible for:
– giving guidelines to regulatory/ technical bodies
– changing regulatory/advisory structures
– individual consent decisions | General public/stakeholders |

| Regulatory/technical bodies (mainly technical expert but with some stakeholder involvement) | Responsible for:
– advising Ministers on individual consent decisions
– giving broader advice to Ministers consistent with their terms of reference | Committee on Safety of Medicines*
Advisory Committee on Pesticides†
Veterinary Products Committee†
Advisory Committee on Releases to the Environment†
Advisory Committee on Novel Foods and Products‡
Foods Advisory Committee‡
Advisory Committee on Animal Feedstuffs‡
Advisory Committee on Toxic Substances§ |

Figure 3.2   General framework of the advisory/regulatory bodies in the UK. Strategic/ advisory body having a primary interest in the work: *Human Genetics Commission; †Agricultural and Environment Biotechnology Commission; ‡Food Standards Agency; §Health and Safety Commission. Sources: Cabinet Office (1999) and Government/Research Councils Initiative on Risk Assessment and Risk Management (1999a).

Occasionally, there is no UK-based advisory committee, in which case the administration (an agency or a local authority) takes the decisions. This occurs when determining whether new substances have been properly notified in accordance with EU directives and UK regulations, and is the likely approach when dealing with integrated pollution prevention and control. In these cases, considerable guidance is available, and the flexibility available to the regulator is kept to a minimum.

In the USA, the tradition has been for agencies to evaluate and manage risks from within, with public discussion of draft evaluations and proposals, but without extensive use of expert/stakeholder committees. The principles by which the evaluations are conducted are published in the Federal Register. When so requested by Congress, committees of the National Research Council review these principles. The results of these reviews have been published, and some examples are listed in Table 3.2. This has led to a reduction in the willingness to accept the conclusions reached, and a greater willingness to challenge conclusions. However, the recent Presidential/

Table 3.2 The international nature of toxic risk assessment for regulatory purposes

International	European Union	National
Drugs and veterinary medicines		
ICH	European Medicines Evaluation Agency (CPMP)	Medicines Control Agency Committee on Safety of Medicines
	European Medicines Evaluation Agency (CVMP)	Veterinary Medicines Directorate Veterinary Products Committee
Food issues		
World Trade Organisation		
Codex Alimentarius Commission (WHO/FAO)	EU Scientific Committee on Food	Food Standards Agency (and Advisory Committees)
JECFA (food additives and contaminants) JMPR (pesticides residues)		
Pesticides		
	EU plant protection products EPPO	Pesticides Safety Directorate Advisory Committee on Pesticides
United Nations Environment Programme	OSPAR	UK DEFRA
Chemicals management		
Organisation of Economic Co-operation and Development (Existing chemicals) (New chemicals) (Test methods) (Good laboratory practice)	EU 'competent authorities' meeting EU Advisory Committee for OELs	National 'competent authority' ACTS and WATCH

Note
ACTS, Advisory Committee on Toxic Substances; CPMP, Committee on Proprietary Medicinal Products; CVMP, Committee on Veterinary Medicinal Products; DEFR, Department for Environment, Food and Rural Affairs; EPPO, European Plant Protection Organisation; ICH, International Committee on Harmonisation; JECFA, Joint Evaluation Committee on Food Additives; JMPR, Joint (FAO/WHO) Meeting on Pesticide Residues; OEL, occupational exposure limit; OSPAR, Oslo–Paris accords; WATCH, Working Advisory Group on Toxic Chemical Hazards.

Box 3.1 Some UK bodies concerned with toxicological risk assessment.

Department of Health
Consumer products
Dangerous pathogens   Advisory Committee on Dangerous
  (jointly with HSC/E)   Pathogens
General policy on health issues   Many advisory committees

Medicines Control Agency
Human medicines and vaccines   Committee on Safety of Medicines
Good laboratory/manufacturing
  practice

Food Standards Agency
Food additives   Foods Advisory Committee,
Food contaminants   committees on carcinogenicity,
                                         mutagenicity and toxicity
Novel foods and processes   Advisory Committee on Novel Foods
                                         and Processes
Food contact materials
Meat hygiene
Additives in animal feeds   Advisory Committee on Animal Feeds
Technological animal feed additives

Department for Environment, Food and Rural Affairs
Pesticides Safety Directorate
Plant protection products   Advisory Committee on Pesticides

Veterinary Medicines Directorate
Veterinary medicines   Veterinary Products Committee
Zootechnical feed additives

Department for Environment, Food and Rural Affairs
Environment Agency
Air Quality   EPAQS
Water quality, including action limits
  for discharges
Waste
Land quality/contaminated land
Releases to the environment   Advisory Committee on Releases to
                                         the Environment

Department of Transport, Local Government and the Regions
Health and Safety Commission/Executive
Occupational exposure limits   Advisory Committee on Toxic
                                         Substances
Dangerous pathogens   Advisory Committee on Dangerous
                                         Pathogens
Biocides   Biocidal Products Committee
Major hazards   Advisory Committee on Major
                                         Hazards

Health and Safety Commission/Executive and DEFRA/Environment Agency
New substances
Existing chemicals
Genetically modified organisms   Advisory Committee on Genetic
                                        Modification

Home Office
Animal welfare (animals subjected to
  scientific procedures)   Animal Procedures Committee

Notes
Based on Government/Research Councils Initiative on Risk Assessment and Toxicology
(1999a), reformulated to allow for the 2001 changes to Government departmental
structures.
DEFRA, Department for Environment, Food and Local Affairs; EPAQS, Expert Panel
on Air Quality Standards.

Congressional Committee (1997) report indicates that such approaches
should be implemented.

Additional comments

Breach of statute law may result in criminal or civil prosecution. Prosecution
under criminal law requires proof 'beyond reasonable doubt', whereas
prosecution under civil law requires proof to the less onerous standard of
'balance of probabilities'. Normally, prosecution under criminal law is
conducted by the State.

In civil law, it is often the individual seeking to prevent harm or seeking
redress for harm suffered who starts the action [in England and Wales, the
'claimant' (formerly 'plaintiff'); in Scotland the 'pursuer']. Prevention is by
means of injunction (interdict in Scotland). Redress is being sought when
civil litigation is undertaken. Typically, the toxicological risk assessments
required in these circumstances are statements provided by expert witnesses
to help the court in its attempts to judge the issue of whether there is harm,
and, if so, how this harm occurred. The issues are decided on 'balance of
probabilities'.

Administrative law may be invoked when someone believes that the State
has taken an improper decision – in the UK, this is a judicial review. Judicial
reviews can be required when a governmental decision is based on internal
toxicological advice or toxicological advice from statutory or non-statutory
advisory committees. Thus, these decisions can affect toxicologists. As the
aim of seeking to obtain a judicial review is to seek to block or change a
decision by the administration, it is sought much more frequently when
there is a clear separation of legislature and administration. It is therefore
much more commonly sought in the USA.

Chapter 4

Philosophical frameworks for handling risk

For the purposes of this book, risk management essentially covers three things: process safety, product safety and environmental protection. It takes place within legal and organisational frameworks as well as within a philosophical framework. In this chapter, I will examine the philosophical framework through investigating several major aspects of risk. The first aspect is what constitutes the risk. The second aspect is the processes for assessing and managing risks, and the third is the criteria for reaching decisions about risk.

What constitutes the risk?

In Chapter 2, I identified that risk management includes, but is not confined to, setting standards. However, examining the types of standards that are set is a useful exercise when looking at what is declared as the risk. Depending on the stage at which control is being exercised, standards may be 'input' standards or 'intake/uptake' standards. 'Input' standards are concerned with the amounts placed into the medium (air, water, soil or food basket) from a particular source (factory stack, discharge sewer, waste disposal site or individual food). They therefore make assumptions about how the material disperses through the medium – and, if necessary, transfers between media – or on the content of the food basket, as well as assumptions concerning intake and uptake. 'Intake' standards are concentration standards for the medium from which absorption takes place, i.e. for material being inhaled from air or ingested from food or drinking water. Intake standards therefore include assumptions concerning the probable amount that will be absorbed (uptake). 'Uptake' standards are measured in the recipient organism and are based on a measure for the amount actually taken into the body.

Depending on the viewpoint, risk can be risk of introduction of a dangerous quantity of a chemical into a medium or risk of a given level of chemical in the medium (or the organism) resulting in ill-health. If the risk is risk of release to the medium, then the difficulties in estimating the ill-health for a given level of material in the medium are considered as uncertainties in defining the hazard. Engineers and others associated with estimating likelihood and sizes of accidental releases of chemicals to media, or with defining the largest acceptable incidental or intentional releases from an industrial plant through a stack or a sewer, are interested in this type of risk. When that chemical is toxic, the release becomes of interest to toxicologists. Food scientists interested in the maximum residue limits in a foodstuff are also concerned with risk of introduction of too much of the chemical (food contaminant, pesticide, veterinary medicine) into the medium (food).

More often, health scientists are concerned with defining the highest amount that can be present in the medium or the body without significant ill-health occurring. They therefore consider risk to be risk of an end-effect (ill-health) resulting from a given level of exposure to the chemical. In these circumstances, how the chemical came to be present in the medium is a separate question.

Processes for assessing and managing risk

In the UK, the Royal Society set up a study group to examine risk assessment. It reported in 1983. In its report, it separated out the stages of risk estimation and risk evaluation – which together constitute risk assessment – and risk management.

Risk estimation includes:

- the identification of outcomes;
- the estimation of the magnitude of the associated consequences of these outcomes;
- the estimation of the probabilities of these outcomes.

Risk evaluation:

- is the complex process of determining the significance or value of the identified hazards and estimated risks to those concerned with or affected by the decision;
- includes, therefore, the study of risk perception and the trade-off between perceived risks and perceived benefits.

Risk management:

- is the making of decisions concerning risks and their subsequent implementation;
- flows from the risk estimation and risk evaluation.

Clearly, this approach was written with the risk of release to medium very much in mind.

Almost simultaneously, the US National Research Council (1983) produced a report, *Risk Assessment in the Federal Government: Managing the Process*. The latter is the now well-known 'Red book'. It identified the stages of risk assessment and risk management as follows.

Risk assessment is:

- the characterisation of the potential adverse health effects of human exposure to environmental hazards;
- is divided into four steps: hazard identification, dose–response assessment, exposure assessment and risk characterisation.

Risk management is:

- the process of evaluating alternative regulatory actions and selecting among them.

The National Research Council approach is more appropriate to setting health-based intake or uptake standards, and it has been widely adopted for the purposes of setting intake standards internationally. Some recent examples are the definitions used by the World Health Organization (WHO)/Food and Agriculture Organisation (FAO) and the definitions proposed to an OECD/WHO project on harmonisation of terminology (Table 4.1).

Although aimed at different risk scenarios, the Royal Society and the National Research Council approaches are not incompatible. The Royal Society's approach is aimed at risk of release into the medium of a significant amount of chemical and the National Research Council's approach is aimed at risk of end-effect – ill-health arising from exposure to a particular level of chemical in the medium. If applied to risk of end-effect, the Royal Society's 'probability of outcome' is the probability of ill-health occurring for the exposure level. The Royal Society's 'identification of outcomes' and 'estimation of associated consequences of these outcomes', taken together, can be considered as the 'hazard identification', 'dose–response estimation' and exposure assessment of the National Research Council. Hence, the two approaches are compatible, and the overall 'risk estimation' of the Royal Society is, in essence, the 'risk assessment' of the National Research Council.

The major difference between these two bodies is the inclusion of a formally defined 'risk evaluation' by the Royal Society. Risk evaluation was also found to be an essential step in risk analysis when the OECD/IPCS project on harmonisation of hazard/risk terminology attempted to produce an annotated list of terms (Lewalle, 1999). The project called risk evaluation:

[the] establishment of a qualitative or quantitative relationship between risks and benefits, involving the complex process of determining the

significance of the identified hazards and estimated risks to those organisms or people concerned with or affected by them.

The project placed risk evaluation as the first step of risk management, although in explaining the definition it suggested that risk evaluation lies between risk assessment and risk management. However, if the risk management is based solely on 'equity' considerations, then risk benefit has no part to play in the risk evaluation (see next section).

Inclusion of this risk evaluation stage is essential if societal concerns are to be taken into the criteria against which the estimation is set when deciding how to manage the risks. Perhaps the most meaningful approach for a health scientist dealing with the management of end-effects is to adopt the 'Red book' approach, but to include explicitly a 'risk evaluation' stage (Figure 4.1) and, when appropriate, exclude the 'source release' assessment. The inclusion of a 'source release' assessment and a dispersion model into the exposure assessment is required when managing risks associated with inputs into the environment. For food chemicals, the source is the release of a chemical residue in a foodstuff into the food basket, and the dispersion model is the mixing of that foodstuff with other foods in the food basket in order to determine the total intake of residue in the diet.

Criteria for reaching decisions about risk

The risk evaluation stage of risk assessment includes the words 'significance or value of' the hazards and risks 'to those concerned with or affected by the decision'. Thus, before any decision is taken about how to manage a risk, the ways in which risks are perceived need to be taken into account.

The Royal Society Study Group (1983) suggested a regulatory process and control strategy based upon:

- an upper level of risk that should not be exceeded for any individual;
- further control, so far as is reasonably practicable, making allowance if possible for aversions to higher levels of detriment; and
- a cut-off in the deployment of resources below some level of exposure or detriment judged to be trivial.

This process has been adopted and publicised by the UK Health and Safety Executive, first when dealing with risks from nuclear power (Health and Safety Executive 1989, 1992) and major industrial hazards (Health and Safety Executive, 1989), and, more recently, in a discussion document concerned with risks generally (Health and Safety Executive, 1999) for industrial risks. The three regions defined through use of the Royal Society process have been called the 'unacceptable', 'tolerable' and 'broadly acceptable' respectively. This has been expressed diagrammatically in Figure

Table 4.1 Some more recent definitions used in risk analysis

Term	WHO/FAO (1995)	Lewalle (1999)
Risk assessment	The scientific evaluation of known or potential adverse health effects resulting from [foodborne] hazards. The process consists of the following steps: (i) hazard identification, (ii) hazard characterisation, (iii) exposure assessment and (iv) risk characterisation. The definition includes quantitative risk assessment, which emphasises reliance on numerical expressions of risk, as well as an indication of attendant uncertainties.	A process intended to calculate or estimate the risk for a given target system following exposure to a particular substance, taking into account the inherent characteristics of a substance of concern as well as the characteristics of the specific target system. The process includes four steps: hazard identification, dose–response assessment, exposure assessment, risk characterisation. It is also the first step in risk analysis.
Hazard identification	The identification of known or potential health effects associated with a particular agent.	The first stage in hazard assessment consisting in the determination of particular hazards a given target system may be exposed to, including attendant toxicity data.
Hazard assessment/ dose–response assessment	The quantitative and/or qualitative evaluation of the nature of adverse effects associated with biological, chemical and physical agents [which may be present in food]. For chemical agents, a dose response assessment should be performed if the data is obtainable.	The second of four steps in risk assessment consisting in the analysis of the relationship between the total amount of an agent absorbed by a group of organisms and the changes developed in it in reaction to the agent, and the inferences derived from such an analysis with respect to the entire population.
Exposure assessment	The quantitative and/or qualitative evaluation of the degree of intake likely to occur.	

Risk characterisation	Integration of hazard identification, hazard characterisation and exposure assessment into an estimation of the adverse effects likely to occur in a given population, including attendant uncertainties.	Step in the process of risk assessment consisting of a quantitative and qualitative analysis of the presence of an agent (including its derivatives) which may be present in a given environment and the inference of the possible consequences it may have for a given population of concern.
Risk management	The process of weighing policy alternatives to accept, minimise or reduce assessed risks and to select and implement appropriate options.	Integration of evidence, reasoning and conclusions collected in hazard identification, dose–response assessment, and the estimation of probability, including attendant uncertainties, of knowledge of an adverse effect if an agent is administered, taken or absorbed by a particular organism or population.
		Decision-making process involving consideration of political, social, economic and technical factors with relevant risk assessment information relating to a hazard so as to develop, analyse and compare regulatory and non-regulatory options and to select and implement the optimal response for safety from that hazard.

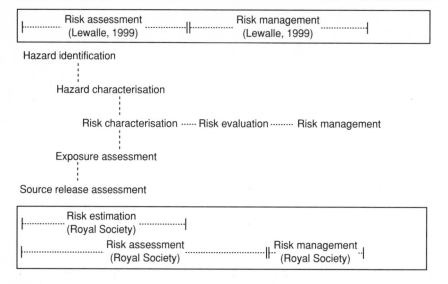

Figure 4.1   Diagram of the process of risk analysis. As the National Research Council did not distinguish the step of risk evaluation, in its terminology risk assessment covers the same ground as the Royal Society's risk estimation.

4.2. What constitutes 'unacceptable', tolerable' or 'broadly acceptable' is a societal judgement and depends on how the public perceives the risk.

The Health and Safety Executive publication *Reducing Risks, Protecting People* (1999) separates the regulatory process into its component criteria. They are:

- an *equity-based criterion*, which starts with the premise that all individuals have unconditional rights to a certain level of protection;
- a *utility-based criterion*, which applies to the comparison between the incremental benefits of the measures to prevent risk or detriment, and the cost of the measures; and
- a *technology-based criterion*, which essentially reflects the idea that a satisfactory level of risk prevention is attained when 'state of the art' technology is used to control risks, whatever the circumstances.

The criterion (or criteria) used will depend on the risk being managed or the standard being set.

Providing that the risk has been fully assessed, the *residual risk* remaining after implementation of the appropriate management procedures should be at least 'tolerable' if not 'broadly acceptable'. However, several elements contained within residual risk may make it necessary to be able to manage the residual risks appropriately. These elements include unidentified or inappropriately assessed risks and inadequately managed risks. The risk

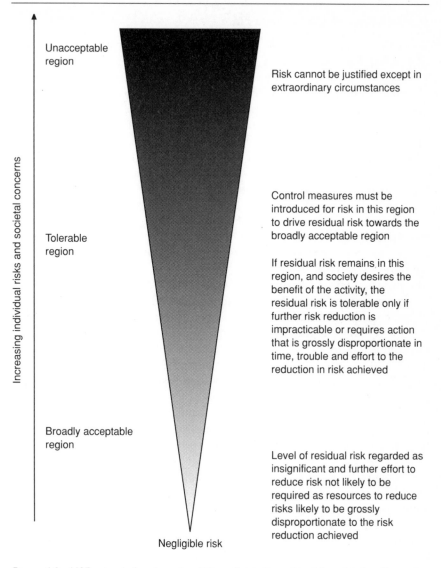

Unacceptable
region

Risk cannot be justified except in
extraordinary circumstances

Increasing individual risks and societal concerns

Tolerable
region

Control measures must be
introduced for risk in this region
to drive residual risk towards the
broadly acceptable region

If residual risk remains in this
region, and society desires the
benefit of the activity, the
residual risk is tolerable only if
further risk reduction is
impracticable or requires action
that is grossly disproportionate in
time, trouble and effort to the
reduction in risk achieved

Broadly acceptable
region

Level of residual risk regarded as
insignificant and further effort to
reduce risk not likely to be
required as resources to reduce
risks likely to be grossly
disproportionate to the risk
reduction achieved

Negligible risk

Figure 4.2   HSE criteria for the tolerability of risk. From Health and Safety Executive
(1999).

management for residual risk will include planning on how to deal with the
unexpected event (in the worst case, emergency planning for disaster
management) and on how to find out the cause and, if necessary, modify the
approach to managing the risks. The latter includes incident investigation
and follow-up research. If the cause includes an element of culpability, the
incident investigation may also furnish evidence to support those seeking
retribution.

Application of these criteria

Many health-based standards are defined in such a way as to indicate that they are seeking to achieve a 'broadly acceptable' or trivial level of risk, sometimes defined as essentially 'zero' risk (Box 4.1). Thus, they are standards associated with equity-based toxicity criteria, and, in the risk evaluation, the evidence concerning toxicity is examined against the appropriate toxicity criterion as the risk evaluation. This applies particularly to UK and international standards associated with the environment (including the UK occupational exposure standard for the workplace environment) and for food chemicals. What happens when this 'broadly acceptable' level of risk is exceeded will depend on the criterion by which the chemical was assessed.

For an intake-based standard set using an equity-based criterion, the need will be to reduce exposure below the standard. When exposure exceeds that standard, the speed with which exposure is reduced to the standard might have to be tempered by practicability. This occurs with air quality objectives, temporary standards using a technology-based criterion. Cost and benefit (the utility criterion) can only apply to the speed with which progress is made towards the equity-based standard. This affects the input standard.

The concept of 'integrated pollution prevention and control' (*IPPC*; now enshrined into EU and UK legislation) includes the ideas of 'best practicable environmental option' (*BPEO*) and best available technique (*BAT*) (mixed utility and technology-based criteria), aimed at minimising inputs which may affect the intake when dealing with emissions of pollutants into the environment.

When risk and benefit can be allowed for, a limit can be set in the 'tolerable risk' region. An occupational 'maximum exposure limit' is set in this region. It carries a continuing duty to reduce exposures to 'as low as is reasonably practicable' (*ALARP*; a mixed utility- and technology-based criterion). Cost and benefit (the utility criterion) can be applied both to the numerical value at which the standard is set and the way in which risks are further reduced. Similarly, the concept of 'integrated pest and pesticide management' (*IPPM*), whereby crop pests are managed only to the extent necessary to reduce crop loss to an acceptable level and with a minimum of pesticide application, is based on trading the benefit of reducing crop losses against the risk of environmental damage due to application of the pesticide.

Three further factors affect the application of these criteria. The first is the exposure circumstances and how the public perceives them; the second is the type of evaluation process used when carrying out the risk assessment; and the third is the 'precautionary principle', which comes into play when evidence is incomplete and/or inconclusive.

All risk assessment has to take place against a background attitude to health and death, and, in the case of food-based risks, with a background of the risks associated with the underlying climate and agro-ecosystem. This is illustrated in Table 4.2.

Box 4.1 Definitions of standards used in the UK.

'Broadly acceptable' risk/'safe' exposure	
Air quality standard	Standards are the concentration of pollutants in the atmosphere which can broadly be taken to achieve a certain level of environmental quality. The standards relating to quality of air are based on an assessment of the effects of each pollutant on public health. From the discussion in the previous section it follows that standards, as benchmarks for setting objectives, are set purely with regard to the scientific and medical evidence of the effects of particular pollutants on health or, in the appropriate context, the wider environment, as minimum or zero risks.
Acceptable/tolerable daily intake	The amount of a substance in food or drinking water, expressed on a body weight basis ($mg\,kg^{-1}$ or $\mu g\,kg^{-1}$ body weight), that can be ingested for a lifetime without appreciable health risk (notional 'zero' risk).
Occupational exposure standard	This is set at a level that (based on current scientific knowledge) will not damage the health of workers exposed to the risk by inhalation.
Other risk levels	
Air quality objective	Objectives provide policy targets by outlining what the government intends should be achieved in the light of air quality standards.
Maximum exposure limit	These are set for substances which may cause the most serious ill-health effects, such as cancer and occupational asthma, and for which 'safe' levels of exposure may exist but control to those levels is not reasonably practicable.

Note
From Illing (1999a).

There are many attributes of hazards that influence risk perception. Some eleven attributes were described in the 1992 report of the Royal Society Study Group (Box 4.2). Attributes 1–3 and 9–11 in Box 4.2 affect the nature of the risk and are likely to be different for different forms of exposure. Environmental air quality standards and, to a lesser extent, food and drinking water standards are concerned with involuntary exposure, lack of personal

Table 4.2 Different circumstances – different acceptability of risks?

	A Western European state	A Third World state
Life expectancy	70 years	45 years
Food supply	Ample	Occasional crop failures lead to famines
Availability of pesticides	Modern pesticides widely available	Only older, cheaper pesticides available, some of which are no longer used in the First World

Note
A pesticide with carcinogenic properties is unlikely to be still suitable for use in Western Europe, where people are likely to survive long enough to acquire chemically induced cancers. In a tropical Third World country with a plague of pests likely to destroy crops and cause a famine, the likelihood of the only effective pesticide available to farmers causing cancer in 15 or more years' time becomes much less unacceptable in view of the need to survive for the next year.

control over exposure and lack of visible benefit. Occupational exposures are, at least to a limited extent, 'voluntary' and involve personal control over outcome through choice of workplace, number and type of control options available, and the extent of control achievable. In addition, the population 'at risk' excludes the elderly, ill, very young (but not necessarily pregnant or lactating women). When dealing with human medicines, there is a much higher level of control again. These all affect the public perception of the risk, and hence the societal criterion of what constitutes a 'broadly acceptable' risk. When uncertainty factors are used for extrapolation, the size of the uncertainty factors used should depend on how the risk is perceived as well as on straightforward technical factors.

The second factor affecting the application of the above criteria is the evaluation process. When a chemical is subjected to full evaluation by a regulatory authority before use, the authority has to pay special attention to preventing an unnecessarily dangerous substance appearing on the market, i.e. *'gate-keeping'*. There are four possible outcomes for any evaluation: correctly passed for marketing; correctly refused permission to market; refused permission but safe; and given permission but unsafe. To prevent, or minimise, the last effect occurring (false acceptance), regulatory authorities are likely also to err in favour of not allowing perfectly safe products onto the market (false refusal). This is a form of conservatism that will be especially reflected in the risk assessment when using an equity-based criterion, where, as benefit is not being traded against the risk, there is little to encourage acceptance.

The third element is the *'precautionary principle'*. This principle originated as the *'vorsorgeprinzip'*. In the UK Department of the Environment's *Guide to Risk Assessment and Risk Management for Environmental Protection* (1995), this is defined as:

Box 4.2 General (negative) attributes of hazard that influence risk perception.

Item no	Description
1	Involuntary exposure to risk
2	Lack of personal control over outcomes
3	Uncertainty about probabilities and consequences
4	Lack of personal experience with the risk (fear of the unknown)
5	Difficulty in imagining risk exposure
6	Effects of exposure delayed over time
7	Genetic effects of exposure (threatens future generations)
8	Infrequent but catastrophic accidents ('kill size')
9	Benefits not highly visible
10	Benefits go to others
11	Accidents caused by human failure rather than natural causes

Note
From Otway and von Winterfeldt (1982), as quoted in Royal Society Study Group (1992).

> Where there are significant risks of damage to the environment the Government will be prepared to take precautionary action to limit the use of potentially dangerous materials or the spread of potentially dangerous pollutants, even when scientific knowledge is not conclusive, if the likely balance of costs and benefits justifies it.

Although this principle is concerned with risk management, it deals with how risks will be managed when the evidence concerning the risk is incomplete. Removal of the 'to the environment' renders this a general statement on how to handle risk management in the face of uncertainty in the risk assessment. Handling this uncertainty will be dealt with in Chapters 8–11.

'*Life cycle analysis*' is a process that may be used in risk analysis in order to ensure that the risks are covered 'cradle to grave'. Thus, undertaking life cycle analysis may well be a part of the evaluation of the justification for the manufacture and use of a chemical.

Summary

In this chapter, I have identified two points for which risk assessments can be undertaken. One is associated with risk of release to the environment or presence in a foodstuff, and the second is associated with risk of ill-health following exposure to an agent in a given environmental medium (air, water, soil) or the food basket. I have also identified that the process of risk assessment includes a stage – risk evaluation – where there is societal input into criteria against which the risk estimation is set in order to determine the acceptability of a risk. This acceptability will depend on whether equity, risk benefit and/or technologically based processes are being used for the risk assessment. Criteria for identifying whether the regulatory system includes these processes are also given. I identify that both societal risk perception and the regulator's perception of how a risk should be managed can affect the criteria used when deciding on the acceptability of a risk. Finally, we observe that, in order to avoid delay, the 'precautionary principle' may be used when taking management decisions in the face of incomplete or inconclusive evidence.

Chapter 5

The importance of risk perception and risk communication for toxicological risk assessment

In the last chapter, I discussed the idea that there may be a societal input into deciding what are 'unacceptable', 'tolerable' and 'broadly acceptable' risks. This depends on how risks are perceived. In this chapter, I deal with risk perception and with the need to ensure that decisions concerning risk are accepted. Implicit in seeking consensus on how risks are perceived and accepted is a need to communicate about risk.

Risk perception

In the original Royal Society Study Group report (1983), risk was divided into 'objective statistical risk' and 'perceived risk'. *Objective risk* is obtained as a numerical estimate from a risk estimation that could be set against a numerical criterion (the 'broadly acceptable' risk). This is based on the assumption that there exists a non-zero level of probability of occurrence of an accident (or *ill-health effect*) below which the public as a whole is willing to accept the risk. Attempts have been made to identify the non-zero risk of death that is considered to be 'broadly acceptable'; these usually use the annual value of approximately one death per million people exposed that was first proposed by the Royal Society in 1983 as an appropriate value. Attempts to produce tentative values for lesser ill-health effects have not been generally accepted.

Toxicologists and other health scientists may use numerical risk estimates when handling suitable epidemiological data. More often, such data are not available. In the absence of suitable numerical data, 'objective' risk estimates may include expert judgements as substitutes for quantitative estimates. Thus, judgmental processes are being used to derive 'broadly acceptable' risk estimates. Often, these judgements are in the form of numerical statements (of exposure levels constituting 'broadly acceptable' risks) obtained in the absence of statistically derived information. When dealing with a chemical's toxicity, the exposure statement incorporates criteria values for the statistics relating to risk of ill-health (or death) included in uncertainty factors and/or decisions on the acceptability of the 'margin of exposure' (see Chapter 8).

Thus, the ways in which these risks are handled can, at least in principal, be considered as statements relating to objective risk, even though numerical risk values are not identified.

Perceived risk is the combined evaluation that is made by an individual. However, we do not fully understand how this anticipation is represented in the mind in the normal course of living. Not infrequently, the public has a different perception from that of the expert.

If risks are to be successfully managed, then there needs to be some reconciliation between the views of the technical experts (objective risk) and those of the general public (perceived risk).

The description given above for objective risk is based on the 'psychometric paradigm' of risk perception, as set out in the Royal Society Study Group's 1983 report. It is a one-dimensional concept, and Jasanoff (1992) has suggested that there are three propositions included in this analysis:

1 given enough data, experts will generally agree with each other in their risk assessment;
2 the only scientific way to think about risk is essentially in actuarial terms, i.e. in terms of expected annual fatalities or annual injuries from the activity in question; and
3 following implicitly from the other two, that any other way of thinking about risk is possibly wrong, certainly unscientific and perhaps even antiscientific.

Jasanoff (1992) accepted that these propositions represent the biases of analysts trained to think in terms of engineering risk, and scientists concerned with biological effects more readily accept the need for qualitative judgements and the possibility of experts disagreeing.

Social scientists generally are unhappy with this psychometric paradigm. In the Royal Society Study Group's (1992) report, they state that:

> There are serious difficulties in attempting to view risk as a one dimensional objective concept. In particular, risk perception cannot be reduced to a single correlate of a particular mathematical aspect of risk, such as the probabilities and consequences of any event. Risk perception is essentially multidimensional and personalistic, with a particular risk of hazard meaning different things to different people and different things in different contexts. Given the essentially conditional nature of all risk assessments one should accept that assessments of risk are derived from social and institutional assumptions and processes; that is risk is socially constructed.

Slovic (1997) suggests that risk assessment is subjective and value laden. He states that:

Attempts to manage risk must confront the question: What is risk? The dominant conception sees risk as 'the chance of injury, damage, or loss'. The probabilities and consequences of adverse events are assumed to be produced by physical and natural processes in ways that can be objectively quantified by risk assessment. Much social science rejects this notion, arguing instead that risk is inherently subjective. In this view risk does not exist 'out there,' independent of our minds and cultures, waiting to be measured. Instead, human beings have invented the concept *risk* to help them to understand and cope with the dangers and uncertainties of life. Although these dangers are real, there is no such thing as 'real risk' or 'objective risk.' The nuclear engineer's probabilistic risk estimate for a nuclear accident or the toxicologist's quantitative estimate of a chemical's carcinogenic risk are both based on theoretical models whose structure is subjective and assumption laden and whose inputs are dependent on judgement. As we shall see, non-scientists have their own models, assumptions, and subjective assessment techniques (intuitive risk assessments), which are sometimes very different from the scientists' models.

This suggests that societal or political dimensions are associated with determining what a 'broadly acceptable' risk is.

The way in which a risk is expressed can affect how the risk is perceived. Box 5.1 sets out ten ways of expressing the risk of death. Alternative ways of expressing these risks – each of which, in isolation, may be considered objective – may result in different views concerning acceptability. A classic case is deaths from coal-mining in the USA between 1950 and 1970. When expressed as deaths per ton of coal extracted, coal-mining becomes much less risky because of higher productivity, but when expressed as deaths per employee it becomes marginally more risky. It is fairly clear which measure the employer or government official will prefer (deaths per ton of coal extracted) and which measure the union leader will choose (deaths per thousand employees)!

Factors such as uncertainty, dread, catastrophic potential, controllability, equity and risk to future generations, voluntariness and immediacy of effect are incorporated into the risk equation by the public (Marris *et al.*, 1997; Slovic, 1997; Langford *et al.*, 1999). For man-made hazards, this can be addressed as 'how well is the process (giving rise to the hazard) understood, how equitably is the danger distributed and how much of it is assumed voluntarily?' (Health and Safety Executive, 1999). There may be both individual concerns and societal concerns (Box 5.2). When managing human medicines, societal concerns are dealt with through the licensing procedure, and individual concerns are examined at the doctor–patient interface when deciding which of the licensed drugs is the most appropriate for the patient.

It becomes perfectly possible for subgroups or individuals within a

Box 5.1 Ten ways of expressing risk of death.

- Per million people
- Per million people and within a given distance of the source
- Per unit of concentration
- Per site or industrial plant
- Per ton of toxic substance releases
- Per ton of toxic substance absorbed
- Per ton of chemical produced (placed on the market)
- Per million pounds (money) of product produced
- Loss of life expectancy associated with exposure to the hazard
- Loss of quality-assured life years of expected life

Note
The first nine ways of expressing risk of death have been reformulated from Slovic (1997). In reality, once born, death is inevitable. Thus, all except the last two methods measure premature death due to the agent. The last two are measures of how premature that death might be.

Box 5.2 Different types of concern.

Individual concern
How individuals see the risk from the hazards affecting them and the things they value personally. Although individuals may be prepared to engage voluntarily in activities that often involve high risks, as a rule they are far less tolerant of risks imposed on them and over which they have little control, unless they regard the risk as negligible. They may also be willing to live with a risk they do not regard as negligible if it secures them or society certain benefits. However, they would want such risks to be kept low and clearly controlled.

Examples: risks to the individual arising from participating in dangerous sporting activities; risks from cancer (to patient, to nurse) that arise from the use of cancer-treating therapeutic agents.

Societal concern
The risks or threats from the hazard that have an impact on society as a whole. This type of concern is often associated with hazards that give rise to risks which, were they to be realised, could provoke a sociopolitical response.

Examples: Potential environmental risks that may arise from the release of genetically modified organisms.

Note
Based on Health and Safety Executive (1999).

population to have different levels of understanding of the process of risk analysis and different attitudes to risk (Langford *et al.*, 1999). 'Worldviews (social, cultural and political attitudes) influence people's judgements on risk issues (Slovic, 1997). Several attempts have been made to classify groups of individuals in respect of 'worldviews' and attitudes to risk (Box 5.3 and Figure 5.1). The conclusion must be that different groups will have very different attitudes towards toxic risks as well as different perceptions of what constitutes a 'broadly acceptable' risk.

In Chapter 4 it was suggested that there is a risk evaluation stage in risk assessment. This risk evaluation needs to take into account differences in the ways that risks are perceived. The social scientists' multidimensional approach to how risks are perceived emphasises that risk assessments are not based on a purely technical paradigm. There is a need to deal with the societal or political dimensions associated with defining the 'broadly acceptable' criterion, and this is conducted within the 'risk evaluation'. Indeed, there may be a family of such criteria, depending on how individuals perceive risk and the circumstances surrounding exposure.

Eleven attributes have been described in the 1992 report of the Royal Society Study Group. Attributes 1–3 and 9–11 in Box 5.4 affect the nature of the risk and are likely to be different for different forms of exposure. Environmental air quality standards and, to a lesser extent, food and drinking water standards are concerned with involuntary exposure, lack of personal control over exposure and lack of visible benefit. Occupational exposures are, at least to a limited extent, 'voluntary' and involve personal control over outcome through choice of workplace, number and type of control options available, and the extent of control achievable. In addition, the population 'at risk' excludes the elderly, ill, very young (but not necessarily pregnant or lactating women) (Illing, 1999a). When dealing with human

Box 5.3 Risk perception and world view.

Fatalism
I feel I have very little control over risks to my health – whatever will be will be.

Hierarchy
Decisions about health risks should be left to experts – command flows down from authority, obedience flows up.

Individualism
In a fair system, people with more ability should earn more – we like to do our own thing untrammelled by government or other constraints.

Egalitarianism
If people were treated more equally, we would have fewer problems - power and wealth should be more evenly distributed.

Technological enthusiasm
A high technology society is important for improving our health and social well being.

Note
From Slovic (1997).

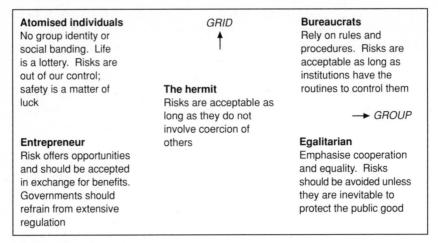

Figure 5.1 Cultural prototypes and their attitudes to risk. Based on a review by Renn (1998).

Box 5.4 General (negative) attributes of hazards that influence risk perception.

Item no	Description
1	Involuntary exposure to a risk
2	Lack of personal control over outcomes
3	Uncertainty about probabilities and consequences
4	Lack of personal experience with the risk (fear of the unknown)
5	Difficulty in imagining risk exposure
6	Effects of exposure delayed over time
7	Genetic effects of exposure (threatens future generations)
8	Infrequent but catastrophic accidents ('kill size')
9	Benefits not highly visible
10	Benefits go to others
11	Accidents caused by human failure rather than natural causes

Note
From Otway and von Winterfeldt (1982), as quoted in Royal Society Study Group (1992; groupings not present in the original).

medicines, there is a much higher level of control again. These all affect the perception of the risk, and hence the societal criterion of what constitutes a 'broadly acceptable' risk.

Thus, subjectivity penetrates risk assessments at every level, from the initial structuring of a risk problem to deciding which end-points or consequences to include in the analysis, identifying and estimating exposures, choosing dose–response relationships, evaluating the risk and so on (Slovic, 1997). Lobbying organisations exploit differences of view concerning risk in order to propagate the idea that the risk manager's view of the risk and how it should be managed is wrong and the lobbyist's particular view should be the consensus view within society. Essentially these organisations are trying to break trust in the risk manager's judgements. Trust is fragile; it is difficult to build up and easily destroyed. Good communication on risk matters is important and participation in the decision-taking process may be valuable. The way in which a risk is described matters (Box 5.5) and careful consideration needs to be given to the language used to communicate about risks (see below). Broad consensus needs be sought in order to ensure that a risk is 'broadly acceptable'.

Box 5.5 Difficulties in communicating risk.

Message problems
- Deficiencies in scientific understanding, data, models and methods resulting in large uncertainties in risk estimates
- Highly technical risk analyses that are unintelligible to lay persons

Source problems
- Lack of trust in responsible authorities
- Disagreements among scientific experts
- Limited authority and resources for addressing risk problems
- Lack of data addressing the specific fears and concerns of individuals and communities
- Failure to disclose limitations of risk assessments and resulting uncertainties
- Limited understanding of the interests, concerns, fears, values, priorities and preferences of individual citizens and public groups
- Use of bureaucratic, legalistic and/or technical language

Channel problems
- Selective and biased media reporting that emphasises drama, wrongdoing, disagreement and conflict
- Premature disclosure of scientific information
- Oversimplification, distortion and inaccuracies in interpreting technical risk information

Receiver problems
- Inaccurate perception of levels of risk
- Lack of interest in risk problems and technical complexities
- Overconfidence in one's ability to avoid harm
- Strong beliefs and opinions that are resistant to change
- Exaggerated expectations about the effectiveness of regulatory actions
- Desire and demand for scientific certainty
- Reluctance to make trade-offs among different types of risk or among risks, costs and benefits
- Difficulties in understanding probabilistic information related to unfamiliar technologies

---

Note
From Cohrssen and Covello (1989).

Risk communication

If there is a social dimension attached to the evaluation of risks and their subsequent management, and this depends on how the public perceives risk, then there is a need to reconcile the conclusions of the technical specialist, the risk manager and the public. At national governmental level, the legislation concerning risk and its management is aimed at providing systems that are accepted by the general public as, at least in democracies, the general public elects its legislature. Communicating about risk and about risk evaluations is essential if the technical assessment is to be properly framed and accepted. Good communication also leads to better compliance with any proposed management procedures.

Risk communication is any purposeful exchange of information about risks. It is the conveying or transmitting of information among interested parties about levels of health or environmental risks and about decisions, actions or policies aimed at managing or controlling health or environmental risks. Interested parties include government agencies, industry and the unions, the media and lobbying organisations, scientific and professional bodies, communities and individuals. Communication takes place through a variety of channels, and ranges from warning labels on chemical bottles through information sheets and the news and television to public meetings, focus groups and polling. The media often serve as transmitters and translators of information, and may amplify as well as constrict public perceptions of risk.

A framework to describe risk communication and its impact on a risk-managing organisation is described by Kasperson *et al.* (1988). The framework is known as the 'social amplification of risk', and is illustrated in Figure 5.2. This framework accounts in a general sense for the different interpretations that individuals and groups will have on hazardous events. The framework, although plausible, is very difficult to test empirically (Royal Society Study Group, 1992).

Cohrssen and Covello (1989) divided communication problems into four groups:

1 deficiencies in scientific understanding;
2 source problems;
3 channel problems; and
4 receiver problems.

Box 5.5 summarises these problems.

Feedback between receiver and source seems to play an important role in this type of communication. There is interplay among psychological, social and political factors. Slovic (1997) suggests that members of the public and experts can disagree about risk because they define risks differently, have different worldviews, different affective experiences and reactions, or

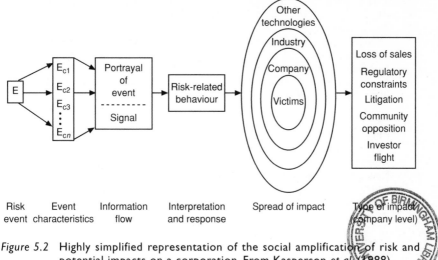

Figure 5.2 Highly simplified representation of the social amplification of risk and potential impacts on a corporation. From Kasperson *et al.* (1988).

different social status. Also, the public often rejects what it views as the 'scientist's' risk assessments because of a lack of trust, although the reality is that a transmitter's interpretation of the scientist's opinions is what is being rejected.

If you trust a risk manager, communication is relatively easy. If trust is lacking, no form of communication will work. Trust is fragile. It takes time to build up and it can be destroyed in an instant. Trust-destroying events are more visible and carry greater weight than trust-building events. Sources of trust-destroying news are often seen as more credible than sources of trust-building news. The media tend to give greater weight to news events that destroy trust, and, of course, lobbying organisations (special interest groups) use their own specialists to communicate concern or distrust and to fan the flame of distrust.

Risk communication in practice

There is, therefore, a need to communicate in order to ensure trust is established and maintained. Guidelines are frequently enunciated, setting out the means by which Government bodies should communicate. Two examples of this are the US Environment Protection Agency's (EPA) 1988 'Cardinal rules of risk communication' (Box 5.6) and the somewhat more succinct principles contained in the Interdepartmental Liaison Group on Risk Assessment's (ILGRA) 1998 commissioned report 'Risk communication: a guide to regulatory practice' (Box 5.7). Language is clearly important, and thought is required concerning the language used to communicate about

Box 5.6 EPA's 1988 'cardinal rules'.

1   *Accept and involve the public as a legitimate partner*
Demonstrate your respect for the public and your sincerity by involving the community early, before important decisions are made. Make it clear that you understand the appropriateness of basing decisions about risk on factors other than the magnitude of the risk. Involve all parties that have an interest or a stake in the particular risk in question.

2   *Plan carefully and evaluate performance*
Begin with clear, explicit objectives. Evaluate the information you have about risks and know its strengths and weaknesses. Classify the different subgroups among your audience, and aim your communication at specific subgroups. Recruit spokespersons who are good at presentation and interaction. Train your staff, including technical staff, in communications skills; reward outstanding performance. Wherever possible pretest your messages. Carefully evaluate your efforts and learn from your mistakes.

3   *Listen to your audience*
Do not make assumptions about what people know, think or want done about risks. Take time to find out what people are thinking: use techniques such as interviews, focus groups and surveys. Let all parties interested in an issue be heard. Recognise people's emotions. Let people know that you understand what they said, addressing their concerns as well as yours. Recognise the 'hidden agendas', symbolic meanings and broader economic or political considerations that often underlie and complicate the task of risk communication.

4   *Be frank, honest and open*
State your credentials, but do not ask or expect to be trusted by the public. If you do not know an answer or are uncertain, say so. Get back to people with answers. Admit mistakes. Disclose risk information as soon as possible (emphasising any appropriate reservations about reliability). Do not minimise or exaggerate the level of risk. Speculate only with great caution. If in doubt, lean towards sharing more information, not less, or people may think you are hiding something. Discuss data uncertainties, strengths and weaknesses, including those identified by other credible sources. Identify worst-case estimates as such, and cite ranges of risk estimates when appropriate.

5   *Co-ordinate and collaborate with other credible sources*
Take time to organise all interorganisational and intraorganisational communications. Devote effort and resources to the slow, hard work of building bridges with other organisations. Use credible and authoritative intermediaries. Consult with others to determine who is best able to answer questions about risk. Try to issue communications jointly with other trustworthy sources, such as credible university scientists, physicians, trusted local officials, and opinion leaders.

6   *Meet the needs of the media*
Be open with and accessible to reporters. Respect their deadlines. Provide information tailored to the needs of each branch of the media, e.g. graphics and other visual aids for television. Prepare in advance, and provide background

---

material on complex risk issues. Follow up on stories with praise or criticism, as warranted. Try to establish long-term relationships of trust with specific editors and reporters.

7   *Speak clearly and with compassion*
Use simple, non-technical language. Be sensitive to local norms in such areas as speech and dress. Use vivid, concrete images that communicate on a personal level. Use examples and anecdotes that make technical data come alive. Avoid distant, abstract, unfeeling language about deaths, injuries and illnesses. Acknowledge and respond (both in words and with actions) to emotions that people express – anxiety, fear, anger, outrage and helplessness. Acknowledge and respond to the distinctions that the public views as important in evaluating risks. Use risk comparisons to help put risks into perspective, but avoid comparisons that ignore distinctions that people consider important. Always try to include a discussion of actions that are under way or can be taken. Tell people what you cannot do. Promise only what you can do, and be sure to do what you promise. Never let your efforts to inform people about risks prevent you from acknowledging – and saying – that any illness, injury or death is a tragedy.

Note
From Cohrrsen and Covello (1989).

health risks. Numerical risk values are generally regarded as not easily understood, so relating numerical values to terms such as 'high', 'moderate', 'low', 'very low' and 'negligible' has been suggested. The use of visual information and comparative information, such as comparisons with size of community, has also been proposed (Calman, 1996; Calman and Royston, 1997). Although governments have set up these principles for risk communication for their use, they are equally applicable to risk communications emanating from commercial organisations.

So far, risk communication has been seen largely as one-way risk communication – making digestible that information being passed from the expert or the risk manager to the general public and obtaining information from the general public to assist in that aim. This may be seen as 'spin doctoring' or, if too crude and one-sided, the production of propaganda. More recent work (Presidential/Congressional Commission on Risk Assessment and Risk Management, 1997, vol. 1; Royal Commission on Environmental Pollution, 1998; Health and Safety Executive, 1999) emphasises that communication is multidirectional as well as multidimensional.

The Presidential/Congressional Commission stated that:

> Involvement of stakeholders – parties who are concerned with or affected by the risk management problem – is critical to making and successfully implementing sound, cost effective, informed risk-management decisions.

Box 5.7 ILGRA's 1998 'Guide to regulatory practice' (ILGRA, 1998).

---

1   *Integrate risk communication and risk regulation*
    The aims of risk communication should be:
    • to enable effective participation and/or representation of all interested
      and affected parties in making decisions about how to manage risks;
    • to support the most effective possible implementation of risk management
      decisions.

2   *Listen to 'stakeholders'*
    Regulatory bodies should identify and engage with all those interested in
    and affected by each risk issue. They should seek to understand their
    attitudes to risk and risk control measures. Their views and preferences
    should be incorporated into policy and practice. Where practical and
    appropriate, those affected should be involved in, or empowered to take,
    decisions about risk and their control

3   *Tailor the messages*
    Government messages and communications about risk should be tailored
    to their audience and purpose. Particular attention should be paid to:
    • engaging and demonstrating empathy with the audience;
    • displaying openness and responsiveness to audience emotions, fears
      and concerns;
    • demonstrating credibility, competence and commitment and purpose;
    • Articulating the benefits of proposed and/or alternative options for
      the audience.

4   *Manage the process*
    • Clear, well-defined risk communication management processes and
      procedures should cover setting goals, allocating responsibilities, planning,
      implementing, monitoring and evaluation.

And

'Stakeholders' typically include groups that are affected or potentially
affected by the risk, risk managers, and groups that will be affected by
any efforts to manage the source of the risk.

The Royal Commission on Environmental Pollution suggested that:

Values should be articulated at the earliest stage possible in setting
standards and developing policies.... The Public should be involved in
the formulation of strategies rather than merely being consulted on
already drafted proposals.

In *Reducing Risks, Protecting People* (Health and Safety Executive, 1999),
the Health and Safety Executive (HSE) outlines its procedure in implementing
and modernising health and safety legislation as:

1   deciding whether the issue is primarily one for the Health and Safety
    Commission (HSC)/HSE;

2   defining and characterising the issue;
3   examining the options available for addressing the issue, and their merits;
4   adopting a particular course of action for addressing the issue, informed
     by the findings of 2 and 3 above, and in the expectation that, as far as
     possible, it will be supported by stakeholders;
5   implementing the decisions;
6   evaluating the effectiveness of actions taken and revisiting the decisions
     and their implementation if necessary.

It is not difficult to discern the similarities in the approach outlined by the
Presidential/Congressional Commission and the Health and Safety Executive.

Implicit and explicit decisions concerning criteria for a broadly acceptable risk

The Royal Commission on Environmental Pollution (RCEP), in its twenty-
first report, states:

> When environmental standards are set or judgements made about
> environmental issues, decisions must be informed by an understanding
> of people's values.

And, the report 'The setting of safety standards' (HM Treasury, 1996)
declares that:

> It is unsatisfactory for public (or other) prejudices to be smuggled into
> policy through apparently technical decision formulae by means of, for
> example, numerical factors imposed subjectively by technical experts
> to reflect supposed ethical or societal concerns.

This leads to the question 'how do we obtain an "understanding of people's
values"' or, put another way, take 'public or other prejudices' (societal
judgements) into the decision-making process. The RCEP identified focus
groups, citizens' juries, consensus conferences and deliberative polls as
methods for articulating values. The difficulties with this procedure are:

1   How are 'articulated values' transcribed into criteria (numerical or
     descriptive) against which to judge evidence of ill-health?
2   How can the evidence be transcribed into a form suitable for setting
     against the criteria?
3   How can transparency be maintained?

The alternative is to deal with the values implicitly, through involvement
of bodies capable of making societal as well as technical judgements when
taking decisions. This is a form of 'stakeholder involvement', as defined by

the Presidential/Congressional Commission on Risk Assessment and Risk Management (1997, vol. 1). If the decision-taking bodies contain a balanced representation of stakeholders, then stakeholders are involved in the decision and the required societal judgements have been embedded into the decisions. It also means that transparency of process is maintained, even if judgements concerning how the evidence fits the criteria and what the criteria are have not been differentiated into their component parts. This is one possible reason why, at least in the UK, membership of official bodies such as the Health and Safety Commission and its Advisory Committees and the Food Safety and Standards Commissions is decided after seeking nominations from stakeholders.

Summary

How risks are perceived critically affects risk assessment and risk management, whether for toxic risks or for any other type of risk. Risk perception has been divided into 'objective' and 'subjective' risk. 'Objective risk' is based on a psychological paradigm and actuarial approaches to annual likelihood of death or injury. 'Objective' risk assessments may be numerical or quantitative, or may depend on technical judgements. Most toxic risks are assessed judgementally, using uncertainty factors and technical experts. 'Perceived risk' depends on public perception and can differ from that of experts. Social scientists see the public's perception of risk as multidimensional and personalistic and that it depends on how the risk is defined and that factors characterising the risk, such as 'dread' affect this perception. The public's perception is not homogeneous, there are different levels of understanding and attitudes to risk and there is a potential for lobbying groups to exploit differences in attitudes. If 'objective' risk and 'perceived' risk are to be reconciled, a consensus opinion must be sought.

The aim of risk communication is to seek consensus, and hence better compliance with risk-management procedures. Risk communication is multidimensional, multifaceted and multidirectional. Media often transmit information imperfectly. There may be deficiencies in the information, the source, the channel or the receiver. One theory concerning the media is that of the social amplification of risk, and one key element in this transmission of information is trust. There are implicit as well as explicit ways by which a problem (toxicological or otherwise) can be articulated, a 'broadly acceptable' risk defined, and suitable risk-management procedures developed. Explicit ways involve a wide variety of communications and information-seeking techniques, including stakeholding, 'focus groups', citizens' juries, consensus conferences and deliberative polls. 'Stakeholding' is also a means of seeking implicit agreement.

Part II

The principles and practice of toxic risk analysis

Chapter 6

Introduction

Royal Society and National Academy of Sciences

In Chapters 2 and 4, definitions of risk assessment and risk management were introduced and I discussed the two major documents, one from the UK Royal Society and the other from the US National Academy of Science, which have influenced risk assessment throughout the world. Although the two approaches are not incompatible, they are very different. It is possible to produce a synthesis, the process shown in Figure 6.1. Chapters 2, 4 and 5 emphasise the contribution of society to the framing of questions about risk and to risk evaluation and management, as well as the importance of the risk evaluation to the overall risk assessment. Chapters 7–12 concentrate on the technical aspects of toxicological risk assessment, but from time to time will refer back to these societal contributions to the process.

Chapter 3 deals with legislative systems involved in risk management. Toxic risks may be assessed in order to deal with public concerns, policy development and the development and application of legislation associated with toxic risks. Both 'permissioning' and standard setting may be required. The chapters that follow are concerned with how toxic risks are estimated or assessed.

Before dealing with detailed risk assessments, it is necessary to consider two more definitions, those for individual risk and societal risk, and how they impinge on risk management. In Jones (1992), *individual risk* is:

> The frequency at which an individual may be expected to sustain a given level of harm [for our purposes ill-health or death] from the realisation of specified *hazards* [for our purposes, exposure to an agent].

And *societal risk* is:

> The relationship between frequency and the number of people suffering from a specified level of harm in a given population from the realisation of specified hazards.

Societal risk is concerned with human populations. When dealing with other organisms, the term *population risk* is used to cover a similar risk.

One difference between individual risk and societal risk is that, while individual risk is universal, societal risk is tied to population, and therefore to a geographic area. Even when the individual risk to people living 1 km from an installation such as a nuclear reprocessing plant, a chemical manufacturing plant or an oil rig is the same, the societal risk from locating the installation in a big city with a high population density is very much greater than it is in a remote area or in the middle of the North Sea.

In Chapter 2, we distinguished among source, pathway and receptor, and hence 'input', 'intake' and 'uptake' standards. Both individual and societal (or population) risk are usually associated with permissioning concerning sources, such as location (land-use planning), operation (safety cases) and emissions ('inputs'). Normally, only individual risk is considered when dealing with human receptors, as happens when examining widely dispersed materials (e.g. agrochemicals, veterinary products, consumer products), and 'intake' and 'uptake' standards. This leads to differences between toxic risk assessments for major industrial hazards and other clearly definable point sources of exposure and for other purposes. Societal risk (associated with human health) and population risk (associated with environmental pollution) may conflict with one another. In areas with a high population, locating away from dense human populations can, and often does, mean locating in the few remaining wilderness areas, and these are likely to be considered as environmentally sensitive.

When dealing with toxic risks, a full risk assessment will involve both hazard and exposure, as shown in Figure 6.1. The hazard is the toxicity, and is identified by assessing information derived from structure–activity reports, experimental studies and human experience. These involve essentially technical judgements. The aim is to identify the types of toxicity likely to be seen if excessive exposure occurs, and the dose–response relationship for these effects. In order to move from hazard to risk, the dose–response curve has to be compared with patterns of exposure. The risk characterisation that results from this process may be expressed numerically, as a probability, but is far more likely to be expressed as a narrative statement, perhaps accompanied by one or several numerical values. In the risk evaluation, this estimate is set against acceptability criteria and decisions (judgements) made concerning the acceptability of the particular proposal. The acceptability criteria should be societally derived (see Chapters 4 and 5), even when applied by technical specialists. Often, they are not clearly enunciated. The management procedures follow on from the risk evaluation.

When dealing with permissioning, exposure levels may have to be predicted or there may be some evidence concerning them from experience gained in testing. For standard setting, the maximum exposure level that is acceptable is the exposure level sought initially. There may be little need to

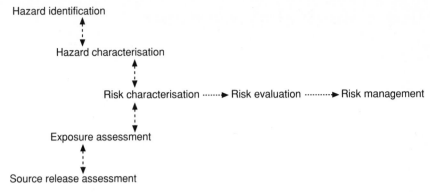

Figure 6.1 Diagram of the process for undertaking a full toxicological risk analysis. This diagram is based on information given in Chapter 4.

define closely the criterion concerning acceptability if exposure levels are never likely to rise to criticality. However, if actual or expected exposures are not well below any clearly acceptable level, the decision ceases to be purely technical. A societal judgement may be required concerning the actual criterion used, and it will need to be clearly defined using an appropriate mechanism. Alternatively, there will need to be some means of evaluating the risks involving both the technical specialists and those affected by the decision. How this can be undertaken was discussed in Chapters 3 and 5.

Chapter 7 will examine the general principles of toxicity assessment and the sources of information on toxicity. The detailed evaluation methods for toxicity and exposure, respectively, for human health will be covered in Chapters 8 and 9, and Chapter 10 will deal with the special case of toxicity for major hazards. Environmental pollution will be covered in Chapters 11 and 12. Chapter 11 will concentrate on the more localised effects, Chapter 12 on global effects.

Chapter 7

Toxicological assessment

General principles

In Chapter 6 we examined what the toxicological assessment is. In essence, it is a hazard assessment, seeking to identify the potential of a chemical to cause various forms of ill-health, and seeking to characterise it, in large part by defining the dose–response relationship. In practice, this is a complex exercise, as effects may be stochastic (all or none) or severity of effect may increase with dose. This is discussed further below.

Two possible procedures are used to translate this information on hazard into information on risk (the risk characterisation). The first is to measure or model exposure levels, set them against the dose–response curve, and determine a 'margin of exposure'. Judgements concerning whether the relationship meets some criterion of acceptability are a part of the risk evaluation and this, in turn, leads to risk-management decisions (Figure 7.1). The second procedure is to take the dose–response information and set it against a predetermined criterion derived from the risk-management system associated with the standard in order to declare what the maximum level of exposure (the standard) should be (Figure 7.2). In practice, this is the 'uncertainty factor' approach and the criterion used depends on the philosophical basis underlying the risk-management procedure. In Chapter 4, we identified 'equity', 'utility' and 'technology' as bases for criteria. In addition, the way in which the information is set against the criterion can depend on the circumstances surrounding the risk-management procedure. This will be discussed further below.

'Conservative' or 'best estimate' – 'gatekeeping', precaution or prediction?

The first pointer that needs checking when deciding how to handle toxicity information is the circumstances surrounding the risk-management process. The risk management may be aimed at preventing unnecessarily dangerous chemicals from entering the market, as with many 'licensing' procedures. In these circumstances, there are four possible outcomes to a licensing process:

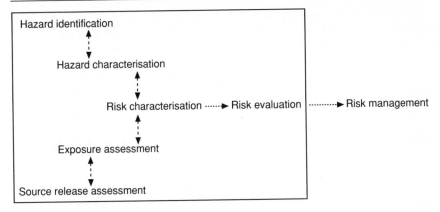

Figure 7.1 The process of toxicological risk assessment as defined by the Royal Society (1983), but using the stages of risk estimation from the National Research Council (1983). This box contains all the elements of a toxicological risk assessment. In the 'margin of exposure' approach the risk evaluation is distinguished from the risk characterisation, and the risk assessment is that defined by Lewalle (1999).

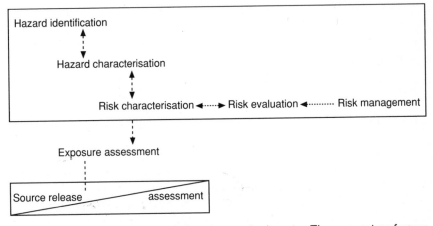

Figure 7.2   The approach to intake/uptake standard setting. The uncertainty factors used to produce the standard (the maximum acceptable exposure) depend on the role of the standard in the risk-management process and on the societal values incorporated into the risk evaluation; the process does not clearly distinguish risk characterisation and risk evaluation.

1   licence granted correctly;
2   licence granted to an excessively dangerous compound;
3   licence refused correctly;
4   licence refused to a sufficiently safe compound.

Outcome 2 may well result in comments questioning the adequacy of the functioning of the body taking the decision. In order to prevent outcome 2, most regulatory bodies (which may be governmental agencies or 'in-house' advisors within large, often multinational organisations) will tolerate a bias that could result in an excess of outcome 4. Outcome 4 is likely to be undetectable because of lack of further development of the compound. Agencies, etc., in seeking to keep dangerous compounds off the market, act as 'gatekeeper'. When acting cautiously, they are acting 'conservatively'. This is especially likely when dealing with purely equity-based standards where there is no need to maintain a realistic relationship to utility-based criteria.

Information may be a problem when conducting toxicological risk assessments. Especially when setting limits in the absence of a licensing procedure or seeking to eliminate use of a compound, acquisition of additional data may take a long time or be prohibitively expensive. Decisions may need to be taken in the absence of data. In these circumstances, the 'precautionary principle' could apply. For environmental risks, the principle has been stated in the form:

> Where there are significant risks of damage to the environment the Government will be prepared to take precautionary action to limit the use of potentially dangerous materials or the spread of potentially dangerous pollutants, even when scientific knowledge is not conclusive, if the likely balance of costs and benefits justifies it.
>
> (Department of the Environment, 1995)

Clearly, it can be adjusted to cover health effects and risk management by other organisations.

This principle can be applied strictly, i.e. taking precautionary management action based on 'worst case' assumptions whenever some information concerning risk is absent and unobtainable within a reasonable time period, or more leniently, taking precautionary action on the assumption of 'best estimate' of what may be occurring. It can also be applied to the need for further testing, particularly if that testing involves long-term studies in animals. A stricter interpretation is likely when a government agency is dealing with a licensing process and data have to be obtained and paid for by the applicant. A more pragmatic approach is likely when there is no applicant and the research has to be funded internally, either by a government or by another organisation.

It is quite easy to apply several 'worst case' assumptions and achieve unrealistic answers. For example, if one assumes a 'worst case' as 1 per cent of the population [probability (p) = 0.01] and applies it three times – say at the dose–response curve, at the exposure measurements and at the level of the model used to derive an input standard – a 1 per cent (10^{-2}) probability has become a one in a million (10^{-6}) probability. Hence, inferences drawn from the 'best estimate' are likely to be very different from those drawn from the 'worst case'. Even if the same process is used to derive estimates concerning toxic risks, the outcome can vary widely, depending on the assumptions used when processing the data.

Even though multiple 'worst cases' may be appropriate to a licensing procedure, where conservative, gatekeeping approaches can be adopted, 'best estimates' are probably more useful when dealing with predictions concerning disaster management, and hence allocation of resources to deal with disasters. Which assumption to make, and when, must depend on the circumstances surrounding the risk and the way in which the risk is being perceived. The choices and the reasons behind them should be clearly stated. These choices may be called policy decisions, but they depend on how society views risk and the risk-management process. They are societal judgements associated with the risk evaluation.

Information sources

Evidence for toxicological risk assessment comes from structure–activity relationships, test reports of laboratory studies, epidemiological studies and case reports. The information may be in the form of publications in the scientific literature or may be presented as test reports. A wide range of effects can be studied, and the studies undertaken should reflect the risk management needs for which the assessment is being performed. Risk assessments should be iterative. Initial assessments are often very simple and use cautious assumptions; these assessments are then refined to the extent necessary to ensure that they are suitable for the purpose. This purpose should be to evaluate the risks, it may lead to identification of requirements for further data and/or a programme of activities aimed at managing the risks.

Predictive testing and *post hoc* studies

In the past, the prime source of information was peer-reviewed articles in the scientific literature. Clearly, with a new substance it is unlikely that there will be much information in the literature. When an older substance is being used in a new role, it is unlikely that the literature will contain all the desired information, and much of the information available is likely to come from studies that would no longer be considered satisfactory. Thus, predictive studies will be required before placing the substance on the market, and post-marketing follow-up studies can be used to supplement the predictive information. The post-marketing studies should confirm that the predictive studies were correct and can provide information on effects not detectable in predictive studies. With the advent of internationally agreed auditing procedures (good laboratory practice, etc.) and standard test protocols, well-written test reports are probably more useful than peer-reviewed papers, although they may be difficult to retrieve. As they are likely only to be available from the sponsor of the test, they are unlikely to be entered into the databases used for literature searching.

Before undertaking animal testing, it should be possible to undertake paper- and computer-based predictive studies. Computer-based structure–activity studies are becoming more common. Originally, structure–activity relationships were built up by comparing effects (such as lethality or a relevant enzyme activity) with chemical structure (often modelled through octanol–water partition coefficients) for a series of congeneric compounds. When measured values were not available, partition coefficients were calculated from structural parameters. This has led to the 'Topkat' system. Nowadays, there are two further approaches to the problem. 'Rule-based' systems are systems that take rules relating structure (usually of a fragment or a particular group/bonding arrangement) derived from the experience of toxicologists and insert the rule into the system ('DEREK'). How effective the rule is in determining whether an effect will occur is tested using a selection of chemicals (ideally not those used to derive the rule) with known results for the property being examined. The new chemical structure is then examined and type of effect and probability of occurrence determined. The most recent developments are in 'neural network-based' systems in which the system develops the information linking structure to effect. Thus, more sophisticated structural information may be used. As yet, these systems are only considered acceptable for obtaining preliminary information before testing; generally, they are not considered acceptable substitutes for regulatory testing.

Standard protocols are available for conducting many of the tests requiring biological material. In order to eliminate repeated testing to similar – but non-identical – protocols, international agreements have been sought. In the drugs and veterinary medicines field, the body seeking standardisation of protocols is the International Committee on Harmonisation (ICH). For other fields of testing, the Organisation for Economic Co-operation and Development (OECD) undertakes the work. A list of OECD guidelines is given in Table 7.1. Because these standard protocols are based on consensus, they take a considerable time to develop. Up to 10 years is not uncommon when developing a new test. This means that tests can be obsolescent for many years while consensus is sought for the protocol to be adopted for the replacement test.

Conduct of animal tests is subject to ethical considerations. Animal welfare lobbies seek the replacement of testing on live animals, and this is enshrined in legislation in the EU. Progress can be made to the three Rs – replacement, reduction in numbers of animals used and refinement of the test procedures (to minimise any pain and maximise the information gain). Some examples where this has occurred are given in Figure 7.3.

As competence of laboratories can be used as a means of disallowing studies, and there were examples of inadequate behaviour in the 1960s and early 1970s, systems for auditing of studies were developed by regulatory authorities in order to ensure the truth of the reports provided to regulatory authorities. These are the Good Laboratory Practice Guidelines. They originated in the USA, and are now extended through the OECD to cover testing centres world-wide. Essentially, the guidelines are to ensure that the test house has an adequate number of suitably qualified staff, proper facilities and proper procedures for managing and conducting studies. This is achieved through inspection by national authorities. Furthermore, the guidelines require that a proper audit trail is available for test protocols, data and report, and that data have been assessed by an in-house (but otherwise independent) quality assurance unit. If required, the inspecting authority can conduct an audit of the data for a particular study to confirm (or otherwise) the statements in the report. Good laboratory practice is not concerned with questions of scientific validity. Its role is to ensure that the study report accurately states what was done and what the results were, and hence to ensure that all regulatory authorities world-wide can have confidence that the report is an accurate representation of the work undertaken.

Because predictive testing is a 'broad brush' approach, a coarse screen for effects, there will always be subtle effects that cannot be detected predictively. For example, there is no test for respiratory sensitisation currently acceptable to regulatory authorities. Also, there are immunotoxicological and long-term neurotoxicological end-points that are not investigated by current testing procedures. This implies that human experimentation and/or monitoring of exposed populations may be required. However, there are clear ethical limitations to how far one can go in studies on humans, and guidelines concerning human studies include the need for a suitably constituted ethics committee to examine and agree to the intended study and proposed protocol.

With drugs, this means that the human exposure to the drug is staged and initial exposure monitored particularly thoroughly. In general, deliberate exposure is unlikely to occur with other chemicals, although some experiments may be carried out under carefully controlled conditions. Thus, the opportunity has to be taken to maximise the information obtained from incidental and accidental exposures. Hence, *post hoc* studies – studies carried out after introducing the chemical onto the market – may be required. This may be in the form of surveillance for adverse reactions or may be in the form of epidemiological studies.

In the long term, it seems possible that a combination of structure–activity relationship information and information derived from early biomarkers for susceptibility to disease and/or the disease itself may render much of today's animal testing unnecessary.

Table 7.1 OECD test guidelines for chemicals

Physical chemistry	Health effects	Degradation and bioaccumulation (fate and behaviour)	Ecotoxicology
UV/visible absorption spectra	Acute oral toxicity (three tests)	Ready biodegradability	Algal growth inhibition test
Melting point/melting range	Acute dermal toxicity	Inherent biodegradability	Daphnia spp. acute
Boiling point/boiling range	Acute inhalation toxicity	Simulation test – aerobic	immobilisation and reproduction
Vapour pressure	Acute dermal irritation/	sewage treatment	Fish acute toxicity test
Water solubility	corrosion (three tests)	Inherent biodegradability	Fish prolonged toxicity test
Absorption/desorption	Skin sensitisation	in soil	Avian dietary toxicity test
Partition coefficient	Repeated dose oral toxicity:	Bioaccumulation in fish	Avian reproduction test
(n-octanol–water)	rodent, 28-day or 14-day study	(five tests)	Earthworm acute toxicity tests
Complex formation ability	Subchronic oral toxicity:	Biodegradability in sea water	Terrestrial plants growth test
in water	rodent, 90-day study		Activated sludge respiratory
Density of liquids and solids	Subchronic oral toxicity:		inhibition test
Particle size distribution/fibre	non-rodent, 90-day study		Fish early life stage toxicity test
length and diameter	Repeated dose dermal toxicity:		
distribution	21/28-day study		
Hydrolysis as a function of pH	Subchronic dermal toxicity:		
Dissociation constants in water	90-day study		
Screening test for thermal	Repeated dose inhalation		
stability and stability in air	toxicity: 28-day or 14-day study		

Viscosity of liquids
Surface tension of aqueous
solutions
Fat solubility of solid and
liquid substances

Subchronic inhalation toxicity:
90-day study
Teratogenicity
One-generation reproduction
toxicity study
Two-generation reproduction
toxicity study
Combined subacute/reproductive
toxicity test
Toxicokinetics
Acute delayed neurotoxicity of
organophosphorous substances
Subchronic delayed neurotoxicity
of organophosphorous
substances: 90-day study
Chronic toxicity studies
Carcinogenicity studies
Combined carcinogenicity/
chronic toxicity
Genetic toxicity studies (fifteen
tests)

Note
Source: OECD (1981, with amendments).

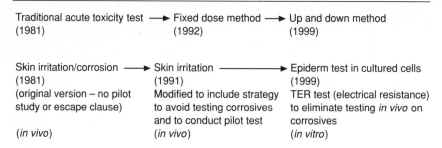

Figure 7.3   Two examples of the introduction of modified tests. It took from 1984 (first publication of 'fixed dose method' proposal) to 1992 (approval of method by OECD) to carry out the development work to demonstrate that it was an acceptable test and to gain acceptance.

Summary

Toxicological assessment is concerned with translation of information on toxic hazard into statements concerning risk. These statements depend on the criteria used and assumptions made concerning attitudes to the information and the criteria in the risk evaluation. 'Conservative' or cautious assumptions ('worst case') tend to be used when 'gatekeeping' or when applying the 'precautionary principle', when others will be responsible for any follow-up. There is a danger that, with multiple applications of 'conservative' assumptions, the overall risk assessment is unrealistic. It may be necessary to identify clearly points at which 'worst case' assumptions are made and points at which 'best estimate' assumptions are used.

Toxicological information comes from the literature and from predictive testing. Literature information may be unsuitable for assessment. Predictive testing includes information on structure–activity relationships and testing using biological materials. These tests are a course screen, and may not detect immunotoxic effects, long-term neurobehavioural effects and other subtle effects. Internationally agreed standard protocols and quality assurance procedures are available for regulatory testing, but take time to develop because of the need for wide acceptance of the procedure. Studies in humans are rare outside the drugs field as exposure is incidental or accidental rather than intentional. Post-marketing monitoring and surveillance of the incidence of ill-health incidents – with, if necessary, follow-up epidemiological studies – is possible. Ethical considerations limit testing in humans and animals. Development of more sophisticated testing may reduce animal usage in the future.

Chapter 8

Evaluation of human health effects
Toxicity

In this chapter, I will cover the examination of studies concerned with defining hazard to humans. Formally, two stages of risk assessment are covered: hazard identification (determining what adverse effects may be caused) and hazard characterisation (determining dose–response or dose–effect relationships for the key effects). Outside labelling requirements for chemicals, hazard characterisation is combined with either risk evaluation or exposure assessment. Normally, the first objective is to examine what constitutes a 'broadly acceptable' risk (a 'safe' exposure) for health effects, either by defining the maximum 'broadly acceptable' risk (standard setting) or by determining whether there is a sufficient margin of exposure that the risk is 'broadly acceptable'.

Information on structure–activity relationships, studies in animals, human case reports, experimental studies in humans and epidemiological studies are all of value in hazard identification and characterisation. These studies are usually carried out iteratively, starting with simple information, possibly from extrapolation and cautious assumptions. If necessary, they lead to a sophisticated assessment in which much more extensive data are gathered and assumptions refined or replaced by actual data. In industry, the process may be divided into investigative toxicology and regulatory assessment, with the former being used to aid decisions concerning whether to develop a new chemical and the latter being undertaken in order to secure regulatory clearance for marketing.

Hazard characterisation

Hazard characterisation is the qualitative, and, where possible, quantitative characterisation of the nature of the hazard associated with a biological, chemical or physical agent, based on one or more elements, such as mechanism of action involved, biological extrapolation, dose–response or dose–effect relationships and their respective uncertainties (Lewalle, 1999). Hazard characterisation is carried out when selecting the labelling requirements for use when supplying industrial chemicals. The 'risk phrases' for use on the label and in safety data sheets are phrases selected on the basis of hazard in order to alert the recipient to possible risks. The EU has set out extensive criteria for translating the results of toxicity tests into risk phrases (Health and Safety Commission, 1999). Otherwise, hazard characterisation is carried out in combination with another phase of risk analysis.

The *dose–effect relationship* is the link between the total amount of a substance administered, taken in or absorbed by a system and the magnitude of a specific continuously graded change affecting it. The *dose–response relationship* is the link between the amount of an agent absorbed by a population and the change developed in that population (Lewalle, 1999). The conventional dose–response curve (Figure 8.1) relates to the statistics associated with stochastic effects. For non-stochastic effects, one can draw a dose–effect curve whereby the severity of the effect increases with increasing dose. This dose–effect relationship obtained in a toxicological study can be converted to a dose–response relationship. If the level of effect seen is fixed, then the statistical distribution associated with that point of the dose–effect relationship constitutes the dose–response curve (Figure 8.1). The dose–response curve also normally applies to epidemiological studies in which the incidence, morbidity or mortality is estimated as frequencies with which certain ill-health criteria are met.

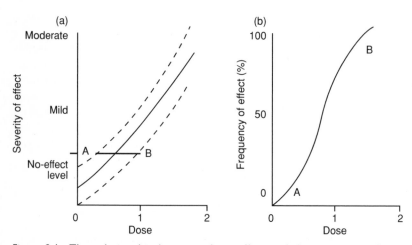

Figure 8.1   The relationship between dose–effect and dose–response for a non-stochastic effect. (a) Dose–effect curve for a non-stochastic effect. (b) Dose–response curve for the level of effect given by the line A to B. A and B refer to the 95 per cent confidence limits for the relationship between the dose and the given level of response.

Dose measurement and scaling factors

When dealing with dose there is a need to consider size of the test and target organisms. Oral or parenteral doses to test species are usually quoted in mg kg^{-1} body weight (b.w.) day^{-1}, except for humans when a simple amount (e.g. mg) may be quoted. Scaling factors are used to convert the absolute values (mg) from one species to another. The simplest scaling factor is body weight, and this is the favoured factor for most regulatory authorities. A number of authors (Calabrese, 1983; Voisin *et al.*, 1990) have suggested that surface area is a better scaling factor, with surface area being approximated by using body weight to the power of 0.7 or two-thirds. Calabrese *et al.* (1992) argued that this scaling factor is independent of the uncertainty factor used for interspecies variation and should be considered independently. However, the convenience associated with the more cautious body weight scaling has led to its continued use.

In inhalation studies, dose is usually measured as concentration and duration of exposure. Thus, there would be two scaling factors, one for body size and one for surface area of the absorbing surface, the lung. In practice, it is assumed that these two scaling factors roughly cancel one another out (Feron *et al.*, 1990).

Stochastic and non-stochastic

One of the essential distinctions encountered in toxicology is that differentiating *stochastic* (presumed all or none) and *non-stochastic* effects (effects for which there is a threshold and severity of effect is related to dose). Stochastic (or pseudo-stochastic) effects include death, carcinogenicity, teratogenicity and immunologically mediated effects. In some cases, there may be a threshold and a dose–effect relationship. However, for genotoxic carcinogens, the working hypothesis is that no threshold exists. In epigenetic carcinogenicity and respiratory sensitisation, a threshold may exist, but the existing methodologies may not allow for its identification in a population. For sensitisation, it may be possible to detect a dose–effect relationship in the individual, but the variation between subjects means that it cannot be satisfactorily detected in a population. With teratology studies, it is generally assumed that a threshold exists and that it can be properly defined during testing. Epigenetic carcinogenesis and teratogenesis are usually treated with the approach described for non-stochastic but severe health effects.

Approaches to non-stochastic effects

The principal approach to determining risk for standard setting is based on determining an amount of a substance at which no adverse effects are seen and applying a factor to that dose (an uncertainty or safety factor). The aim is to extrapolate to a dose (exposure level/duration) that is considered the maximum dose to be 'without risk to health', i.e. a dose that meets the criterion for a health-based 'broadly acceptable' risk or a 'safe' exposure. The alternative approach is the 'margin of exposure' approach. The amount at which no adverse effects are seen (the NOAEL) is compared with the predicted or actual doses or exposure levels (concentration/time) and the ratio between the two values compared. The ratio is the 'margin of exposure'. Judgements concerning the acceptability of the margin of exposure are conducted separately.

The uncertainty factors approach

The uncertainty factor approach takes the hazard identification, hazard characterisation and risk evaluation stages of risk analysis together and derives an exposure statement from the resultant analysis. Assumptions are made concerning both the societal and policy inputs into the criteria for acceptability (as expressed through the uncertainty factors) and the risk-management process for which the exposure statement is being developed. The process is outlined in Figure 8.2.

The overall 'uncertainty factor' procedure can be described using the equation:

$$RfD = \frac{NOAEL \left(\text{or LOAL or BMD}\right)}{\text{Uncertainty and modifying factors}}$$

where RfD is the reference dose, NOAEL is the no observable adverse effect

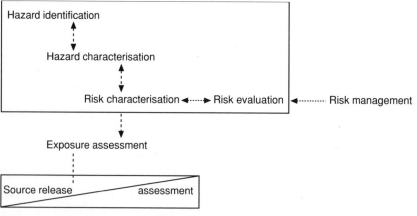

Figure 8.2   The approach to determining risk management for intake/uptake standard setting. The outcome of the process is an exposure assessment, a statement of the maximum acceptable level of exposure.

level, LOAEL is the lowest observed adverse effect level and BMD is the benchmark dose.

These elements are examined more closely below.

The 'no observed/observable adverse effect level' and related parameters

Essentially, conventional toxicological effects are non-stochastic. There is a gradation of severity of effect with dose, from minor disturbances to observations, clinical chemical parameters, through mild and moderately severe pathological changes to, in the worst case, death. The normal approach to toxicological assessment is to determine a 'no observable adverse effect level' (NOAEL) and to use 'uncertainty' factors to convert the NOAEL to a 'safe' dose (exposure level), the 'reference dose' or possibly the proposed standard. Sometimes, a close relation to the NOAEL – such as the 'lowest observed adverse effect level' (LOAEL) or the 'benchmark dose' (BMD) – is used as the starting point for application of uncertainty factors. The benchmark dose is derived statistically, as shown in Figure 8.3.

Originally, the NOAEL was called the no-effect level. Addition of observed (for a particular study) or observable (for a comprehensive review of the information from all the studies on a particular chemical) reflects the dose levels seen in the study or group of studies. It also implies that there is a frequency at which effects may be occurring in the population, but that the frequency is sufficiently low that the effect is not seen in the particular sample

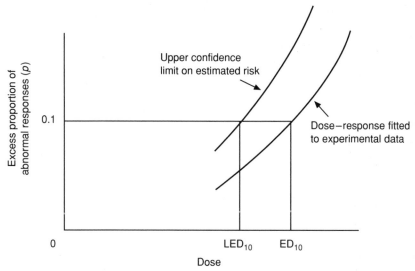

Figure 8.3   The benchmark dose. The benchmark dose is calculated from the upper 95 per cent confidence limit for the dose–response curve at the borderline point just corresponding to 'no-effect:effect' on the dose–effect curve. From this is derived the low ED_{10} (LED_{10}), which is taken as the benchmark dose.

of the population (the test group examined). Given the relatively small size of groups in toxicological studies (five for 28-day studies, ten for 90-day studies, fifty for chronic toxicity or carcinogenicity studies according to OECD protocols), quite high (and unacceptable) frequencies may occur in the population that are not detected in the sample. One reason for the use of uncertainty factors (or for ensuring a suitable margin of exposure is to ensure that the (much lower) highest acceptable frequency of occurrence in the population is not exceeded.

Statistical significance is usually taken, as a minimum, as the 95 per cent probability that the 'null' hypothesis is untrue. There will be a finite number of 'false positives' and of 'false negatives'. False positives (statistical significance where there is really no effect) are usually examined for in terms of biological plausibility, but false negatives (non-significance even when the frequency in the population is high enough to be statistically significant) are much more difficult to detect. Biological plausibility is examined by looking at other measured parameters that might be altered, but not to the point of statistical significance. If there is a dose–effect relationship or related parameters are altered at the same or higher dose levels, then it is more plausible that a real effect was being observed.

Even with the statistical significance implied by the term observed/observable, there is a second question: 'Is the effect seen adverse?' This question is examined in Box 8.1. It shows how complex and difficult it can be to define the NOAEL.

The 'low observed adverse effect level' is often used when a NOAEL is not available. The 'benchmark dose' is an attempt to make use of the statistical information associated with the dose–effect curve. In place of the NOAEL, the upper 95 per cent confidence limit (the one yielding the lowest dose as the benchmark dose) is used as the 'benchmark' (Figure 8.3).

Critical effect and pivotal study

Whichever of NOAEL, LOAEL or BMD is chosen, there then follows a process to select from within all the information available the critical effect and the pivotal study. Usually, there will be several effects that might be the lead effects, dependent on the circumstances surrounding likely human exposure. The critical effect will be that which, under the envisaged exposure conditions, yields the lowest maximum exposure value when the NOAEL (etc.) and uncertainty factors are combined. Thus, it may be necessary to evaluate several end-points before taking a final decision concerning what the critical effect is. The pivotal study is the study from which the NOAEL (etc.) is derived.

Box 8.1 Defining toxic effects at or near the NOAEL and their relevance to humans.

Non-adverse effects are the absence of changes in morphology, growth, development and life span. Furthermore, non-adverse effects do not result in impairment of functional capacity or impairment of the capacity to compensate for additional stress. They are reversible following cessation of exposure without detectable impairment of the ability of the organism to maintain homeostasis, and do not enhance susceptibility to the deleterious effects of other environmental influences. (From IPCS, 1978.)

Effects that may be considered not toxic but deemed normal physiological responses required for the maintenance of homeostasis:

Laxative effects from osmotic or fecal overload.

Liver hypertophy and microsomal enzyme induction from high doses of substances metabolised by the liver.

Decreased body weight gain or caecal enlargement from high levels of non-nutritive substances.

Alterations in kidney weight due to the amount of water being processed.

Decreased growth weight and food consumption related to the dietary administration of unpalatable substances.

However, care must be taken to ensure that they are not automatically dismissed as unimportant. (From IPCS, 1987.)

Evidence not indicative of serious damage to health on prolonged exposure but that needs to be taken into account when determining a no-effect level:

Clinical observations or changes in weight gain, food consumption or water intake, which may have some (minor) toxicological importance.

Small changes in clinical biochemistry, haematology or urinanalysis parameters that are of doubtful or minimal toxicological significance.

Changes in organ weight with no evidence of organ dysfunction.

Adaptive responses (e.g. macrophage migration in the lung, liver hypertrophy and enzyme induction, hyperplastic responses to irritants).

Where a species-specific mechanism of toxicity has been demonstrated.

By implication, these effects may be, but need not be described as, 'adverse'. (From Health and Safety Commission, 1999.)

Uncertainty factors and modifying factors

Uncertainty factors are intended to make allowances for interspecies and interindividual variation, conversion from subchronic to chronic, LOAEL to NOAEL and an incomplete database. Modifying factors are introduced to cover the professional assessment of the scientific uncertainties of the study and the database not explicitly included in the uncertainty factors (Dourson *et al.*, 1996). A list of these technical uncertainty and modifying factors is given in Table 8.1. In addition, societal judgements associated with the criterion for 'acceptability', as applied in the risk evaluation, need to be incorporated into these uncertainty and modifying factors (Illing, 1999a). The factors affecting these societal judgements have already been discussed in Chapters 4 and 5. Only recently has it become recognised that these judgements concerning uncertainty factors should take into account society's attitudes to the type of risk being examined, and hence should not be taken solely by technical experts. There is a societal, as well as a technical, element to the opinion expressed.

Interspecies and interindividual variations

Interspecies and interindividual variation (applied as a single combined factor of 100) were the two uncertainty factors first used when regulating food additives in the 1950s (Lehman and Fitzhugh, 1954). They are now regarded as two key default uncertainty factors for toxic risk assessment (Rubery *et al.*, 1990; IPCS, 1994; Dourson *et al.*, 1996, Government/Research Councils Initiative on Risk Assessment and Risk Management, 1999a,b). The interspecies variation is to account for potential differences between the population mean for one species (the test species) and the population mean for the target species for which the evaluation is being conducted. The target species is usually human, but for veterinary medicines it may be another species such as the cow, sheep, dog or cat and for environmental toxicology it may be a sentinel wildlife species. The initial choice of factor for interspecies variation is usually ten, although this may be varied in the light of the evidence

Table 8.1 List of uncertainty factors

Uncertainty from	Conventional value of factor
Animal to human	10
Human average to sensitive	10
Nature of toxicity	Up to 10
Adequacy of data package	Variable (1–100; 3, 5, 10 preferred)
Adequacy of pivotal study	Variable (3, 5, 10 preferred for LOAEL to NOAEL)

Note
Usually only the first three factors are relevant when there is good predictive animal data (from IPCS, 1994).

available. Renwick (1993) divided this factor into two parts, one relating to toxicokinetics and one relating to toxicodynamics. Originally, he suggested factor values of 3.2 for each part, but this was modified by IPCS (1994) to 4.0 for toxicokinetics and 2.5 for toxicodynamics. If direct evidence is available, this should be substituted for the default factor in question.

Interindividual variation is concerned with the spread of variation. Generally, the factor used is also 10, although that factor is likely to vary somewhat according to the type of population being considered and how completely the population should be covered. This factor can also be divided into two parts, one (of 3.2) for toxicokinetics and one (also of 3.2) for toxicodynamics (Renwick, 1993; IPCS, 1994). The factor is usually claimed to cover 'nearly all' of the relevant target population and has to account for genetic and environmental factors that affect susceptibility. These may be temporary developmental factors affecting children or the elderly or they may be genetically determined factors (such as consequences of immunological differences leading to allergies or consequences of different catalytic capacities of foreign compound-metabolising enzymes leading to differential toxicity) (Government/Research Councils Initiative on Risk Assessment and Toxicology, 1999b). Although Renwick and Lazarus (1998) provide evidence from an analysis of data on drugs confirming the suggestion that the allowance for toxicokinetics in humans will not be satisfactory for all subgroups, Renwick (1998) has suggested that further allowance for infants and children (by a factor of more than ten times) is unnecessary. The factor for interindividual variation may also have to allow for variation in the test population. For many older animal studies, a heterogeneous animal population may have been examined, for modern tests an inbred strain is likely to have been used in order to minimise interindividual variation. If human studies are available, then the way in which the population examined was selected is one of the factors that has to be considered when deciding on the appropriate uncertainty factor.

LOAEL to NOAEL

If the extrapolation is made from a study for which a LOAEL only is available, an uncertainty factor (three, five or ten) may be applied to the LOAEL to allow for the fact that it is not a NOAEL (IPCS, 1994; Dourson, 1996).

Severity of effect

Generally, the NOAEL (or equivalent) is presumed to be for a minor effect or even a small perturbation in a clinical chemical or behavioural parameter. When the nature of the toxicity differs and the effect being examined is severe – as with terata- or non-genotoxic cancers, or when severe pathological lesions are seen without mild effects being examined – then an extra factor of ten may be incorporated (Johnson, 1988; IPCS, 1994; Renwick, 1995).

Duration of study

The NOAEL for a chronic effect is usually derived, if possible, from a long-term repeated dose study. Generally, the longer the dosing period the lower is the NOAEL. This can be accounted for using a conversion factor; Kramer *et al.* (1996) calculated that this factor should be eighty-seven when converting a NOAEL from a subacute (3–6 weeks) study to a long-term NOAEL. Dourson *et al.* (1996) suggest a conversion factor of ten is appropriate when converting from subchronic (usually taken as 3- or 6-month dosing) to long-term NOAEL.

The 90-day repeated dose study (i.e. subchronic) is the study chosen for classification purposes when dealing with chemicals under the European dangerous substances directives (Health and Safety Commission, 1999), thus appropriate adjustments to NOAELs could be required when deciding what label to apply.

Route-to-route extrapolation

In the case of occupational exposure, route-to-route extrapolation from parenteral or oral to inhalation may be a necessity. The effects of parenterally administered doses (complete absorption) may be used as a 'worst case' approximate prediction of what might occur following inhalation exposure (Pepelko and Withey, 1985; Pepelko, 1987; Withey, 1987). The approach used for oral exposure to inhalation – the 'Stockinger–Woodward' approach – assumes that a dose (in mg kg^{-1} for an 80-kg human) causing a toxic effect is completely absorbed and is contained in a volume of air approximating to that breathed during a working day. That volume is often assumed to be 10 m^3 for an 8-hour day, based on the idea that physical effort is expended during work. The very different metabolic capacities of the two 'portals of entry' means that the approach has severe limitations. If sufficient toxicokinetic information is available, then the extrapolation may be valid (Pepelko and Withey, 1985, Pepelko, 1987; Withey, 1987). However, sufficient information on inhalation toxicity *per se* is usually available before adequate toxicokinetic studies are available and the inherent assumptions validated. Generally, this is discouraged (Sharratt, 1988).

Quality of data

Incomplete data are rarely a significant problem when dealing with a regulatory scheme whereby full data are submitted before permission to use is given. When the decision has to be taken on the basis of existing data, as with existing chemicals and food contaminants, then incomplete data may be a problem that is overcome by the application of a variable enlargement (one- to 100-fold) of the safety factor.

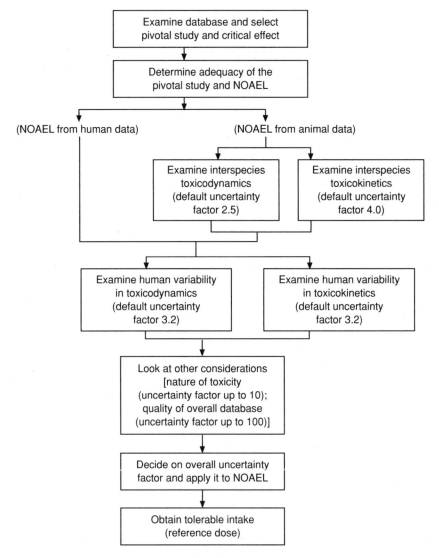

Figure 8.4 Outline of the procedure for applying the uncertainty factors approach. From Illing (1999a); based on IPCS (1994).

The overall procedure

The overall procedure is outlined in Figure 8.4. The final stage in setting the overall uncertainty factor is to apply a modifying factor as a professional assessment of scientific uncertainties of the study and database not explicitly treated elsewhere. Values of 0–10 have been suggested (Dourson *et al.*, 1996). In practice, this modifying factor is a way by which the professional (the technical expert) covers for societal factors that affect the choice of uncertainty factors in the absence of more societally directed input.

Should there be variations in default values for the final uncertainty factor?

Despite the wide variety of uncertainty factors that can be applied, the most common default continues to be the 100-fold factor, increased to 1,000 when a severe effect such as a teratogenic or a non-genotoxic carcinogenic effect is seen. This 100-fold factor is the original factor chosen by Lehman and Fitzhugh in 1954 for application to food chemicals. This is essentially the uncertainty factor associated with an equity, 'gatekeeping', 'broadly acceptable' health-based standard.

Generally, workplace standards developed independently of standards for food additives and contaminants. Much smaller uncertainty factors are usually used for health-based occupational exposure limits such as the UK Occupational Exposure Standard (Illing, 1991a, 1999a; Fairhurst, 1995). The approach used is essentially that employed for the 'Threshold Limit rates of the American Conference of Government Industrial Hygienists'. Although the standard is equity-based, it has to fit into a mixed equity/ utility/technology-based system, thus the conservatism associated with 'gatekeeping' and precaution is absent (see Chapter 4). There are also good technical and sociological reasons why the defaults used for occupational exposure can differ from those used for food chemicals. One technical reason is that the meaning of 'nearly all' is seldom defined further. In reality, there has to be allowance for the type of population affected. Generally, a working population contains very few children, elderly and seriously ill members, whereas the general population includes all of these. There are also sociological reasons (see Chapter 4) associated with the circumstances surrounding the exposure that would indicate that a smaller uncertainty factor would still be appropriate while maintaining that the health-based standard is based on a 'broadly acceptable' risk criterion.

When an occupational exposure level is based on 'tolerable risk', the toxicology will not be the sole determinant for the standard. However, it may be used in conjunction with other factors to determine the exposure level set. Any NOAEL required may be for a serious effect rather all toxic effects, and/or the uncertainty factor might be less than normal because of the higher level of risk considered 'tolerable'. An example of this is the UK Maximum Exposure Limit, a limit derived using utility and technology criteria (Health and Safety Executive, 1999).

Although it may be possible to exclude clearly defined parts of the population when dealing with an occupational exposure standard or a standard for a food additive or contaminant by advising them to avoid the relevant occupation or foods entirely, this is more difficult to accomplish when dealing with environmental exposures. Environmental standards use equity criteria for a health-based 'broadly acceptable' risk. Often, the chemical is already present in the environment, so 'gatekeeping' is not possible and standards may not be so conservative. Developing environmental air quality standards is a comparatively recent phenomenon, thus there is less clarity about default uncertainty factors, although they tend to follow the general pattern described for food chemicals.

The 'margin of exposure' approach

For many regulatory purposes, the 'margin of exposure' approach can be used to determine the acceptability of a toxic risk. In effect, this procedure incorporates hazard identification, hazard characterisation, exposure assessment and risk characterisation into a form of risk estimate (Figure 8.5). The advantage of this approach is that it clearly separates the risk characterisation from the risk evaluation. The disadvantage is the need for some estimate of exposure.

The 'margin of exposure' (MoE) is defined as:

$$MoE = \frac{NOAEL \left(or\ LOAL\ or\ BMD \right)}{Exposure\ level \left(measured\ or\ predicted \right)}$$

If the MoE is less than 1, then it can be concluded that there is a definite risk

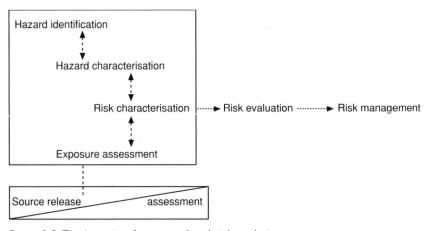

Figure 8.5 The 'margin of exposure' and risk analysis.

of the (ill-health) effect occurring, and the greater the numerical value of the MoE the less the risk of ill-health. Often, the MoE value can be refined iteratively as further information becomes available. The risk evaluation, the decision concerning the acceptability of the MoE, contains the technical decisions associated with uncertainty factors outlined above as well as societal decisions concerning how acceptable the risk is.

Relationship to the psychometric paradigm and probabilistic risk assessment

When the uncertainty factor approach was first developed in the 1950s, risk was examined deterministically (safe/unsafe), whereas most risk assessors now use probabilities when describing risk. A major question is 'how does the uncertainty factor approach to risk assessment fit into the psychometric paradigm and probabilistic approaches currently favoured outside toxicology?' In this approach, the criterion for acceptability is expressed numerically. It is usually expressed as 'risk of death' or risk of cancer and a value of excess risk of 1 in 10^6 (lifetime risk, annual rate) is used as the criterion for the general public). If the social scientists' criticism of this paradigm is correct (see Chapter 4), then society will require more than one criterion, and each criterion will depend on the circumstances surrounding the risk.

In reality, the risk is for foreshortened life or reduced quality of life due to exposure to the chemical. In practice, the risk usually sought is much less than risk of death. Although there is some agreement concerning risk levels for severe, life-threatening effects – including death, the 'dangerous dose' and cancer – for most effects a much lesser ill-health effect, the NOAEL, is required. Sporadic attempts have been made to look at criteria in terms of these lesser effects (Illing, 1991b, 1993; Niemeyer, 1993), but they have not been accepted generally.

When extrapolating using uncertainty factors, the aim is to move down the statistical distribution for the frequency of occurrence of a given level of effect to a statistical value representing a very low frequency. Although theoretically possible (Figure 8.6), this usually involves extrapolation well beyond the actual data and assumptions concerning the linearity of the extrapolation. Should hormesis occur (as for, for example, with vitamins and minerals), the approach becomes difficult. If there is an insufficient gap between the minimum amount required for normal function and the minimum amount at which high dose toxicity occurs, a 'risk minimisation' needs to be attempted by seeking extrapolation from both curves (Figure 8.7). Essentially, this is a move from an 'equity-based' to a 'utility-based' criterion (Chapter 4) for judging risk, and the system chosen has moved from being a pure equity-based system to a mixed system which includes the concept of 'tolerable' risk. A similar mixed system based on 'tolerable'

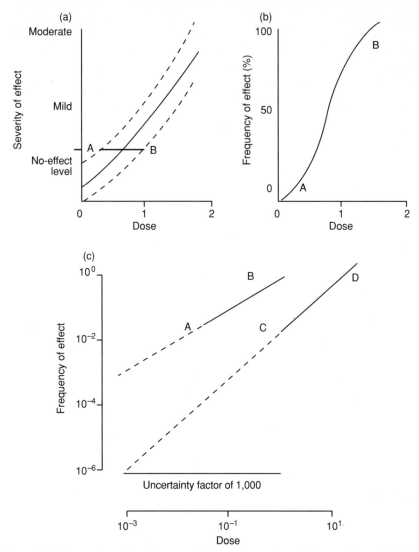

Figure 8.6 How uncertainty factors relate to frequencies of effect and hence criteria for a 'broadly acceptable' risk. (a) Dose–effect curve. (b) Dose–response curve for the level of effect on or just above the NOAEL. (c) The extrapolation to low frequencies of effect likely to be used to represent a 'broadly acceptable' risk ('safe' dose). A and B refer to the positions of the 95 per cent confidence limits. In (c), an uncertainty factor of 1,000 is shown for the effect associated with AB. Note that (b) is a linear diagram and (c) is a log–log diagram and assumes a linear extrapolation for the dose–response relationship. The diagrams are hypothetical. One hundred per cent is a frequency of 1 in 1 (10^0) and 1 per cent is a frequency of 1 in 100 (1 in 10^2, or 10^{-2}). From Illing (1999a).

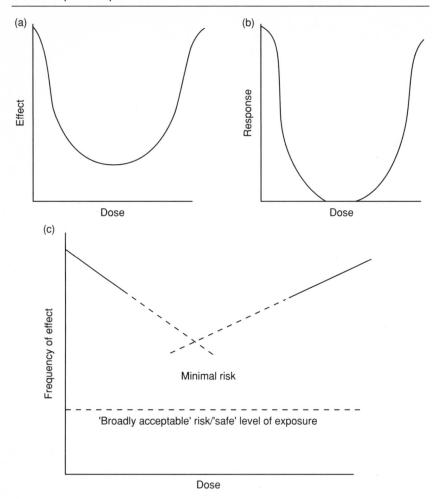

Figure 8.7 The trade-off of risks when dealing with uncertainty and both high-dose and low-dose toxicity. (a) Dose–effect curve for the two effects (assuming both are ill-health). (b) The dose–response curves developed for each effect. (c) The trade-off to minimise the risks. The scales are linear in (b) and the lines are transformed so that linear extrapolations can be carried out in (c). If dealing with a beneficial effect, a similar trade-off is obtained by treating low-dose lack of benefit as harm.

risk is used for drugs. Some are deemed to be an 'unacceptable' risk in all circumstances; for others, the risks (side/toxic effects) are 'tolerable' in order to gain some therapeutic benefit. This is the risk benefit exercise usually conducted when selecting the appropriate therapeutic agent for treating the patient.

Box 8.2 IARC classification of carcinogens (IARC, 1997).

Group 1 – The agent (mixture) is carcinogenic to humans
This category is used when there is sufficient evidence of carcinogenicity in humans. Exceptionally, an agent (mixture) may be placed in this category when the evidence in humans is less than sufficient but there is sufficient evidence of carcinogenicity in experimental animals and strong evidence in exposed humans that the agent (mixture) acts through a relevant mechanism of carcinogenicity.

Group 2A – The agent (mixture) is probably carcinogenic to humans. The exposure circumstance entails exposures that are probably carcinogenic to humans
This category is used when there is limited evidence of carcinogenicity in humans and sufficient evidence of carcinogenicity in experimental animals. In some cases, an agent (mixture) may be classified in this category when there is inadequate evidence of carcinogenicity in humans, sufficient evidence of carcinogenicity in experimental animals and strong evidence that the carcinogenicity is mediated by a mechanism that also operates in humans. Exceptionally, an agent, mixture or exposure circumstance may be classified in this category solely on the basis of limited evidence of carcinogenicity in humans.

Group 2B - The agent (mixture) is possibly carcinogenic to humans. The exposure circumstance entails exposures that are possibly carcinogenic to humans
This category is used for agents, mixtures and exposure circumstances for which there is limited evidence of carcinogenicity in humans and less than sufficient evidence of carcinogenicity in experimental animals. It may also be used when there is inadequate evidence of carcinogenicity in humans but there is sufficient evidence of carcinogenicity in experimental animals. In some circumstances, an agent, mixture or exposure circumstance for which there is inadequate evidence of carcinogenicity in humans but limited evidence of carcinogenicity in experimental animals together with supporting evidence from other relevant data may be placed in this group.

Group 3 – The agent (mixture or exposure circumstance) is not classifiable as to its carcinogenicity to humans
This category is used most commonly for agents, mixtures and exposure circumstances for which the evidence of carcinogenicity is inadequate in humans and inadequate or limited in experimental animals. Exceptionally, agents (mixtures) for which evidence of carcinogenicity is inadequate in humans but sufficient in experimental animals may be placed in this category where there is strong evidence that the mechanism of carcinogenicity in experimental animals does not operate in humans.

Group 4 – The agent (mixture) is probably not carcinogenic to humans
This category is used for agents or mixtures for which there is evidence suggesting lack of carcinogenicity in humans and experimental animals. In some instances, agents or mixtures for which there is inadequate evidence of carcinogenicity in humans but evidence suggesting lack of carcinogenicity in experimental animals, consistently and strongly supported by a broad range of other relevant data, may be classified in this group.

Extrapolation for stochastic effects

Mutagenicity and genotoxic carcinogenicity are the two effects considered as stochastic effects. These are all-or-none effects, and a 'weight of evidence' approach is used in making decisions as to whether a substance is a carcinogen or not and whether the carcinogenic effect is due to genotoxicity or to a non-genotoxic (epigenetic) mechanism. Essentially, this is hazard identification, with the International Agency for Research on Cancer (IARC, 1997) and different regulatory authorities having subtly different schemes and procedures for evaluating the evidence. The definitions and categories used by the IARC are given in Box 8.2. Most schemes deal in terms of known human carcinogens, probable human carcinogens and possible human carcinogens. The IARC has additional classifications involving lack of adequate evidence and evidence suggesting lack of carcinogenesis.

Once the hazard has been identified, assumptions are made concerning mechanism of action. Either it is assumed that there is no threshold or it is assumed that there is a threshold but it cannot be identified on the basis of current knowledge and current experimental capability (Government/ Research Councils Initiative on Risk Assessment and Toxicology, 1999a). The notion of threshold is therefore absent in the approaches used for stochastic effects. Much risk management is based on hazard identification with only limited hazard characterisation, i.e. potency assessment. It is assumed that only the more potent carcinogens are identifiable, and, usually, that deliberate exposure to genotoxic carcinogens is to be avoided. However, in the case of human pharmaceuticals, risk benefit is applicable. Cytotoxic drugs are known carcinogens used to treat cancers. The threat of the cancer that is being treated is much more immediate than that of any cancer caused by the drug used in the treatment.

There are two approaches to assessing the risks of genotoxic carcinogens. Any risk estimation has to include an estimate of potency (hazard characterisation) as well as an identification that the substance is carcinogenic. The difficulty in human risk assessment for carcinogens is the problems associated with extrapolation. Ideally, human epidemiological studies with good quantification and stratification of exposure levels are required for quantitative estimates. These are extremely unlikely to be available. Generally, when available, epidemiological studies yield relatively simple answers (yes/no with a minimum of exposure information). Thus, great reliance has to be placed on animal studies.

The first approach to this problem is pragmatic and is the TD_{50} approach of Peto et al. (1984), based on databases provided by Gold et al. (1984, 1986, 1987, 1990, 1992a). The TD_{50} is defined as 'the chronic dose rate in mg kg^{-1} b.w. day^{-1} which would have the actuarially adjusted percentage of tumour-free animals at the end of the "standard" life span for the species'. Quantitative extrapolation from the animal studies in the database to the human situation has to be conducted cautiously as it needs to be based on

Table 8.2 Models used in quantitative cancer risk assessment

Category	Model	Description
Stochastic (or mechanistic)	One hit	Based on the theory that a single 'hit' (DNA damage/binding at receptor) can initiate an irreversible series of events leading to cancer and the probability of a hit is directly proportional to concentration
	Multi-hit	An extension of the one-hit model which assumes that multiple hits are required to initiate the cancer
	Multistage (Armitage–Doll)	Assumes several random events are required in sequence for the development of a cancer. Transition rates between successive stages are not necessarily equal. The carcinogen affects at least one of the transitions
	Linearised multistage (Hartley–Sielkin)	A special case of the Armitage–Doll model, in which the rates of occurrence of the different changes are all directly proportional to the dose
Tolerance distribution	Weibull Logit Probit (Mantel–Bryan)	The models assume that a population contains a distribution of individuals of different susceptibilities
Time to tumour	Log-normal distribution	Tumours are defined as fatal or incidental and age at death is used as an approximation for time of occurrence of the fatal tumour. Detects differences in time to tumour as well as differences in overall tumour incidence
	Weibull	Based on time to failure for electrical and mechanical components, with ability to represent threshold and concave curves
	Armitage–Doll Hartley–Sielkin	
Biologically motivated	Moolngavkar–Venzon Knudson	Biologically based model. Assumes malignant tumours arise from a single malignant cell and that the malignant transformation of the stem cell is the result of two specific rate-limiting irreversible events that occur during cell division. The model depends on 'birth' and 'death' rates of 'normal', 'initiated' and 'transformed' cells, data that are difficult to obtain

Notes
Stochastic models are loosely compatible with a broad range of experimental observations in carcinogenesis. Tolerance models are based solely on curve-fitting methods.
Based on Committee on Carcinogenicity (1991), ECETOC (1996) and Lovell and Thomas (1996).

an understanding of mechanisms of carcinogenesis at high and low dose (Gold *et al.*, 1992b).

The second approach is probabilistic, and is the preferred approach in the USA. When extrapolating from animal studies, it is necessary to look at a mathematical model for extrapolating to the low levels of exposure that are likely to give the low frequency of cancer occurring required for regulatory purposes. A list of models is given in Table 8.2. In the past, the 'linearised multistage model' using upper bound (95 per cent) estimates has been favoured. Currently, linear extrapolation from the upper bound 95 per cent estimate is used. The linearised multistage model yields a numerical exposure value clearly related to a numerical risk estimate and therefore separates the risk estimation from the risk evaluation and management. It is much criticised (Committee on Carcinogenicity, 1991; ECETOC, 1996; Lovell and Thomas, 1996) as:

- the upper confidence limit is relatively insensitive to changes in experimental tumour incidences and therefore lacks discrimination;
- it is dependent on the highest administered dose rather than on the dose response within the data set;
- there is little or no theoretical (biological) support for the basis of extrapolation.

Even if the maximum likelihood estimate was used in place of the upper confidence limit, the method is still unsatisfactory because the estimate is unduly sensitive to small changes in the data (ECETOC, 1996; Lovell and Thomas, 1996). Some of this criticism may be a translation difficulty between the literate, who believe that numbers convey improper exactitude and precision, and the numerate, who believe that subtle use of words to convey imprecision can lead to misinterpretation and confusion. The latter have some justification, as a survey reported by Woodward and Dayan (1990) indicated that subtle meanings are largely lost in interindividual interpretational differences.

The approach used most often in the UK by regulatory authorities is essentially a pragmatic risk-management system. A 'case by case' basis on 'weight of evidence' approach is followed (Committee on Carcinogenicity, 1991; Maynard *et al.*, 1995; McDonald *et al.*, 1996). Only a vague, descriptive estimate of risk is all that can be achieved. Essentially, the eventual result is that cautious application of uncertainty factors to the 'no expected human effect level', a level at which it would not be possible to demonstrate an effect in epidemiology studies. This is coupled with guidance that exposure should be reduced 'as low as is technically achievable' or 'as low as is reasonably practicable'. In the occupational exposure scenario, a limit may be set, but this carries a requirement to reduce exposure as far as reasonably practicable below that limit. The whole process mixes the technical and societal elements of risk assessment and risk management.

None of these approaches is entirely satisfactory. In the long term, there are two potential approaches that might yield more acceptable results. The first is to obtain toxicokinetic and toxicodynamic information in the test and target species for the relevant compounds and to use these data to carry out the extrapolation between species. If this is coupled with suitable Monte Carlo approaches to population variability, then a reasonable estimate of the risk to humans might be obtained. However, this process is highly data intensive and so can only rarely be used. The second approach is to develop and utilise early biomarkers in humans. This approach is still at an early developmental stage. Thus, there is no quick, simple and reliable procedure for estimating cancer risks from experimental data.

Physiologically based toxicokinetic and biologically based dose–response approaches to extrapolation

Pharmacokinetics has developed as a discipline associated with medicines. Absorption, distribution, metabolism and excretion of the chemical are simulated by equations describing actual physiological processes, and the model behind the equations is based, as far as possible, on the physiological and biochemical structures of the relevant species. The equations describe transport into blood, partition into tissues and enzymatic conversion. These parameters can be measured in a test species, and, by substituting information from the target species, can extrapolated to that target species. These physiologically based pharmacokinetic (or toxicokinetic) approaches to extrapolation have been available since the 1930s, but it was because of useful computer power in the 1970s that it became possible to make more widespread use of them. They were developed initially for anaesthetic gases, and extended to volatile chemicals of occupational interest in the 1970s.

At the same time it is possible to consider modelling the toxicodynamics of a chemical by considering the relationships between toxicological receptor concentration of chemical (in the relevant organ by extrapolation from blood data) and the related effect. When combined with toxicokinetic information, the overall process is known as biologically based dose–response (BBDR) modelling. Toxicodynamic modelling is less advanced, thus there is much less information on how to undertake the work.

Essentially, physiologically based toxicokinetics (PBTK) is undertaken in a series of steps:

- The model is specified, based on the anatomy and physiology of the species of interest and the determinants of disposition and biotransformation for the relevant substance.
- A mathematical description is developed for the biological processes involved. This model includes physical, physicochemical and biochemical constants.
- The model is tested experimentally and refined.

Initial models tend to be overcomplex, and one of the consequences of the experimental testing of the model is its simplification. The model needs to be as complex as is necessary to facilitate accurate extrapolation, yet as simple as possible in order to minimise data requirements.

PBTK and BBDR modelling gives the opportunity to substitute for uncertainty factors when extrapolating between species. When combined with the Monte Carlo models for developing population statistics, they offer the opportunity to substitute data in place of the use of uncertainty factors. However, the vast amount of data required means that this approach will only be rarely used.

Basis of extrapolation

The methods employed for extrapolation for non-stochastic effects can be related to the methods used for quantitative (probabilistic) risk. The 'no observed(able) adverse effects' and uncertainty factor approaches were developed in the days of deterministic risk assessment, but it is quite possible to adapt the rationale for their use to a rationale based on probabilistic risk assessment principles. The uncertainty factor approach is a default approach and physiologically based toxicokinetic and toxicodynamic data can be used to improve the basis of the extrapolation. At the same time, data-rich physiologically based toxicokinetics and toxicodynamics ('biologically based dose response') does permit quantitative estimates of risk. The psychometric paradigm of risk can therefore be shown to underlie this approach to risk assessment, even though the criterion used in the risk estimation has not been clearly stated.

The psychometric paradigm can also be said to underlie both the quantitative cancer risk assessment and the biologically based dose–response approach. However, the sociological basis underlying the 'pragmatic' (or judgemental) approach to carcinogenic risk is more difficult to identify. The lack of scientific confidence in the quantitative cancer risk assessment renders it less acceptable to the scientific community, but it can be clearly set out. The lack of clarity inherent in the pragmatic approach means that there are communication difficulties between the scientific assessors and the public, and hence there is a likelihood of very different perceptions of the risk.

If a purely technical group takes a judgement in which risk assessment and risk management are at least partially integrated, then the criticism can be levelled that there has been no proper societal input into that decision and the decision and process are flawed. One of two approaches is possible. In the first approach, the technical decision is propelled through a political process to determine how acceptable it is to society. In the second approach, representatives of the appropriate societal elements ('stakeholders') participate in the decision. This element of the decision-taking process is discussed in Chapter 5.

Chapter 9

Evaluation of human health effects

Exposure

In Chapter 2, I identified that there are two forms of standard, 'input' standards and 'intake/uptake' standards. 'Input' standards are those relating to inputs into the medium (discharges into air, water or residues in foodstuffs). 'Intake' standards refer to the concentrations in the medium from which absorption occurs, and 'uptake' standards to the amounts in the receiving organism. In this chapter, I examine how the 'reference dose' identified using the procedures outlined in Chapter 8 is transformed into these standards, and how exposure measurements ensure that a standard is feasible and is being adhered to. The first stage is to examine the relationship between reference dose (RfD) and intake/uptake standard.

From reference dose to intake/uptake standard

The risk associated with an intake or uptake standard is the risk relating exposure to end-effect and the stage of risk analysis being dealt with and is shown in Figure 9.1. Setting the standard involves information from the risk characterisation and depends on the risk evaluation, which, in turn, depends on the role of the standard in managing risk. Ensuring the standard is feasible and is adhered to is a part of risk management.

The exposure level chosen as standard depends on the reference dose (RfD). In the conventional theory, the RfD (or doses) should cover all exposures (Government/Research Councils Initiative on Risk Assessment and Toxicology, 1999a). The aim would be to obtain an overall risk assessment for total human exposure to any single chemical that has multiple uses and/or is a ubiquitous environmental pollutant. However, as explained in Chapter 8, the uncertainty factors used for different types of exposure can differ for a variety of reasons. This leads to different RfDs for different circumstances of exposure; thus, it is not realistic to undertake an overall risk assessment based on partitioning a single RfD among the various routes of exposure. Nevertheless, it is possible to consider grouping of exposures with similar risk criteria, such as all exposure from food and drink or all non-occupational environmental exposure. The relevant reference dose has

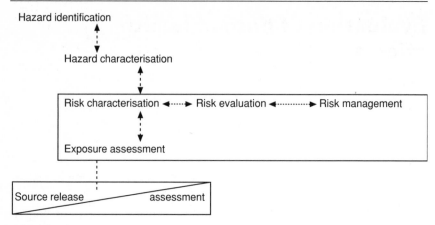

Figure 9.1 Intake/uptake standards and exposure measurements.

then to be allocated on the basis that exposures other than those being considered are not critical to the decision and/or are not likely to change sufficiently significantly that they invalidate the decision.

Exposure assessment (measured exposure or, if not practicable, predicted exposure based on modelled information) is used to indicate whether the standard is practicable, and hence what risk-management strategies may be appropriate. Exposure measurements are also a part of monitoring strategies to ensure that the management strategies are being adhered to.

'Intake' standards

Intake standards are based on the amount of material in the medium (outdoor, indoor, workplace air, drinking water, food – as acceptable/tolerable daily intake) that can be taken in. Standards are expressed as quantities in the medium, thus assumptions are made concerning amounts of air breathed and duration of exposure, amount of food eaten and/or amount of water drunk. Generally, a health-based standard is set at or around the value of the reference dose, and, generally, only in the case of food and drinking water is the contribution of each to the reference dose considered. If separate standards are set for each medium (food and water), each standard usually assumes that the amount present in the other medium is the maximum permitted amount; as, generally, the amounts actually present will be less than those permitted by the standard, the assumption is 'conservative'.

The next problem that needs ascertaining is whether the proposed standard can be adhered to. If data are available, then they are the best source of information. However, existing data are likely to be absent prior to marketing. Because monitoring data are expensive to collect, unless there is a specific reason why the data should have been collected, they are also absent for most other chemicals. In the absence of measured data, models may be used to estimate likely exposure levels. Although not used for formal standard setting, they are valuable as a screening tool for determining the acceptability of risks. One such model is the 'predictive operator exposure model' (Pesticides Safety Directorate, 1986, 1992). This model is used in the UK process for licensing plant protection products for predicting exposure of sprayers, takes account of contamination from handling the concentrated product when preparing spray, and contamination during spraying. The former depends on product-specific data, the latter on spraying technique-specific data. A second model, used for workplace exposure, is 'EASE', outlined in *Risk Assessment of Notified New Substances* (Health and Safety Executive, 1994). It uses information on the physical properties of the substance during processing to describe the tendency to become airborne, and incorporates into the assessment the use patterns of the substances, from closed systems to widely dispersive uses, and pattern of control, from full containment to direct handling. This leads to a series of exposure fields for which ranges of exposure have been described, based on information collected in the UK. For dermal exposure assessment an additional parameter, level of contact, is included in the system. These systems need to be updated regularly to keep them in line with industrial practice.

Monitoring to ensure that an 'intake' standard is being adhered to can be by measurement in air, water or food. For air monitoring, what matters is the air breathed in, thus personal sampling in the breathing zone is more relevant than background monitoring. However, personal sampling is more difficult as the sampler must be portable. Thus, personal sampling is more frequently used for workplace sampling and background sampling trends to be used for monitoring the wider environment. Personal sampling usually involves adsorption of the chemical onto a filter, transfer of the filter to a laboratory, and desorption and analysis of the chemical by conventional analytical procedures. Background air sampling also includes continuously recording direct measurement equipment. Food analyses involve extraction of the chemical from the food and measurement by conventional analytical techniques. Standard assumptions concerning absorption (usually complete), amount of air inhaled (standard weight, exercise state and breathing rate) or total amount of food eaten (from dietary exposure studies) and water drunk ($2 \, l \, day^{-1}$ for adults; $1 \, l \, day^{-1}$ for a 10-kg child; $0.75 \, l \, day^{-1}$ for a bottle-fed infant; Fawell and Young, 1999) are used to link 'intake' and 'uptake'.

'Uptake' standards

Uptake standards and guidance values include 'biological exposure indices' of the American Conference of Governmental Industrial Hygienists, the 'biological monitoring guidance values' of the UK Health and Safety

Executive and the corresponding values of the Deutsche Forshungsgemeinschaft (Wilson, 1999). These are forms of biological monitoring, and measure total uptake – either a level of parent compound or metabolite – in or near a biological matrix. Suitable media in which to conduct measurements include exhaled breath, urine or blood. Time of sampling is important as allowance has to be made for the toxicokinetics associated with the chemical and sampling medium. A second form of biomonitoring, biological effects monitoring, may also be employed. Biological effects monitoring is used to give an early indication of potential health effects, and involves the measurement of biochemical, immunological or physiological responses to hazards. Although health-based guidance values will depend on the same factors as those relating to intake standards, they will be based on different measurement parameters. Outside medicines, monitoring using these 'biomarkers' is restricted to a small number of substances.

Relationship between intake, uptake and effect

If the intake standard is for the dominant contributor to the overall uptake, then the intake and uptake measures should correlate. However, the clarity with which that relationship can be derived will depend on interindividual variation in toxicokinetics and the contributions from other routes of exposure. For example, an air intake standard will be unlikely to correlate with uptake measure if there is significant and variable skin absorption taking place as a consequence of deposition of splashes of the material on hand and forearm. Correlation of an uptake standard with 'NOAEL' is very difficult, given the complexities of dose–effect relationships and the imposition of uncertainty factors on the NOAEL.

From reference dose or intake standard to input (and input standard) or beyond (or vice versa)

In this approach, risk is taken as risk of release to the environment or risk of presence in the food, rather than risk that the amount in the environment/food sample will cause the end-effect (ill-health). In these circumstances, the intake standard or reference dose is part of the definition of hazard and its attendant uncertainties are uncertainties in defining the hazards. Thus, what constitutes the risk has changed from that used when dealing with input standards.

This approach is intended to cover the circumstances when source release assessment and exposure assessment are required for risk estimation (Figure 9.2). The initial approach used for this section is to consider how the reference dose (RfD) or intake standard relates to the input standard, the maximum/median residue level/limit for the contents of a chemical in a foodstuff or

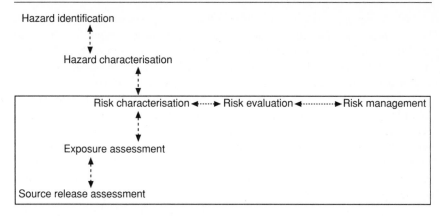

Figure 9.2 Input standards and exposure measurements.

emission/discharge standard for emission to air or discharge to water. The problem may be approached in the reverse direction by determining whether the likely input from a particular source will result in breach of an intake standard or reference dose. The latter approach is often adopted when dealing with risks arising from industrial pollution sources and leachate from waste disposal sites, and for assessing the potential risks arising from the redevelopment of contaminated land sites. In all cases, exposure assessments have three elements: identifying the source of the chemical; identifying the dispersion pattern through the environment or food supply; and selecting a suitable harm criterion against which to set the concentrations derived from the exposure assessment. The dispersion pattern is that required for normal use or for foreseeable minor accident/misuse.

Environmental exposures

Environmental exposure may arise from discharges from industrial plant and waste disposal sites. These are essentially point sources of pollution. While direct control of current discharges – including waste disposal – may be possible, control historically may have been less adequate. Thus, reclamation of contaminated land etc. may become necessary. This can be expensive, and polluted land should only be used for redevelopment once adequate remediation has taken place. Nevertheless, sometimes development took place before controls were established, thus remediation has to be conducted afterwards.

Other sources of pollution may include pesticides and agrochemicals, and anthropomorphic sources. In many cases these will be, in effect, diffuse sources. Control of these sources may be more difficult.

Release of pollutant may be covenanted (intentional or incidental) or uncovenanted (accidental).

When dealing with environmental releases, an exposure assessment will be required. It should take into account the mechanisms, probability, duration and magnitude of the exposure to a hazard. When dealing with discharges, it is assumed that a release of known size will occur, but when dealing with major accident hazards (Chapter 10) the probability of an event and the size of the release have to be predicted. For toxic hazards, the receptors will include humans, but the models will also be applicable to ecotoxic hazards (Chapter 11). The evaluation needs to extend from initiation to the point at which harm becomes manifest. It can involve a source of the hazard in the receiving environmental medium or direct release of the pollutant to the receiving medium. It also has to account for movement through the medium, and hence advective transport and distribution to the point at which exposure occurs. The models and processes used will depend on the sources. The basis of the models will depend on the medium. That for air dispersion will depend on wind and weather. Soil and ground water dispersion patterns can be modelled similarly, but will depend on adsorption onto particles and directions and rates of flow of surface and ground water under various weather conditions. Hydrological river/estuary/coast-specific models will be needed when examining discharges through the sewer, treatment works and river/estuary/coast. Multimedia transport and distribution processes between recipient medium and other indirect media may affect dispersion. When dispersion patterns from several sources overlap, the discharge limits have to be set so that the overall input standard is sufficiently low that the concentration in the medium (air/surface or ground water/soil) into which the emission/discharge is being permitted does not exceed the concentration described in the intake standard. When allocating limits, the assumption is often made that the other discharges are actually at their limit; if this is not the case, the limits allocated are essentially 'conservative'.

In addition to understanding the natural processes of dispersion, it can be necessary to consider transport of wastes to landfill sites or to incinerator. Waste control includes regulatory processes to ensure that industrial waste materials are disposed of successfully. Classification as hazardous waste depends on the classification of hazard undertaken for industrial chemicals. Conditions are then applied as to how the material may be disposed of that depend on the hazards recognised. The exercise is largely hazard based.

Food exposure

Residue limits in individual foods also need to be set using some form of modelling if the overall acceptable/tolerable daily intake is not to be exceeded. There are several approaches to the assessment of dietary exposure. The approaches to dietary exposure estimation are shown in Box 9.1. Generally, estimates can be refined using improved data (Box 9.2).

Food consumption information is obtained from nutritional surveys, total

Box 9.1 Approaches to assessing dietary exposure (based on Rees, 1999).

Methods for 'average' values for exposure
'Per capita' approach. The dietary exposure estimate reflects the average amount of a substance available to a member of the population usually over an average year. 'High consumers' can have exposure that is several times the average.

Total diet survey approach. The dietary exposure estimate is based on an 'average' diet derived from studies of households. This method does not describe the possible distribution of exposures by individual consumers.

Methods for more specific information
Critical groups approach. The dietary exposure estimate is based on a group of individuals assumed to have the highest exposure. Subgroups of the population may be classed as a 'critical' group because of their geographic location, higher susceptibility or consumption or greater exposure to other, non-food sources.

High-level approach. The dietary exposure estimate is based on the top end of a distribution of a representative sample of consumers. The underlying assumption is that the dietary habits giving rise to dietary exposure higher than the 97.5 percentile are unlikely to be maintained over a significant part of an individual's lifetime.

Worst-case approach. The exposure is estimated using worst-case assumptions: for example, all relevant food in the diet contains the chemical at a maximum level. If such an estimate falls below the level of concern, then it usually means that further work is not required.

Box 9.2 Methods used for estimating exposure to chemicals in food.

FIRST ESTIMATE	
Consumption data	*Residues data*
(Single point method)	(Cheapest source)
Model diets	Maximum levels in standards
Regional diets	Monitored levels
National diets	Monitored levels
Household/individual diets	As consumed levels
(Probabilistic methods)	(Best quality)
BEST ESTIMATE	

---

diet studies, duplicate diet studies and studies on special age groups and groups with particular dietary habits. Estimates of food additive intake are usually made from information on the use levels required to achieve a given technical effect. Surveys of chemical residues in individual foods include information on environmental pollutants, food contact materials, natural toxins and pesticides, and veterinary product residues in individual foods can be used to develop estimates of intake for these chemicals.

Modelling is being developed for use in exposure estimation. Distribution data models estimate exposure by taking into account the statistical distribution of consumption and the distribution for concentrations of chemical in the individual foods. The mean value and the standard deviation describe chemical concentration, and a maximum value for chemical concentration is incorporated. Typical weights of the foods samples from which the chemical was determined are incorporated into the model. Duration data models are used when examining exposure for shorter or longer time periods than those used for the actual collection of the food consumption data. They are particularly useful for examining chemicals that exhibit acute toxicity. The dietary survey information is modelled over time by assuming that the daily dietary habits are repeated randomly over the time period.

'Best estimates' and 'worst cases' may be used when dealing with residue levels in individual foods. Generally, 'best estimate' is used when dealing with agricultural pesticide residues, and is obtained from field trials. However, 'worst case' (in this case exemplified as the 97.5 percentile intake value) is used for food additives and contaminants. Toxicokinetic data are used to develop withdrawal times for veterinary medicines. The withdrawal time is set such that 95 per cent of the carcasses should meet the residue level standard, so there may be an additional application of 'worst case' estimation in this instance. 'Worst case' estimates are essentially conservative.

Consumer products

Assessment of exposure for consumer products, other than those for which more specific procedures apply, is based on use (ECETOC, 1994; Health and Safety Executive, 1994). The methods are capable of refinement (ECETOC, 1997), and should be refined in the light of monitoring data as and when data become available. Both normal use and reasonably foreseeable misuse are covered. The aim is to use 'worst case' only as a preliminary calculation and 'reasonable worst case' as the normal calculation. 'Reasonable worst case' covers normal use patterns, including cases where consumers may use several products containing the same substance, as well as the majority (claimed 95 percentile) of foreseeable extreme use and misuse.

There are separate algorithms for each route of exposure (Box 9.3). The algorithms depend on assumptions contained in product use scenarios. Typical product use scenarios include those for cosmetics and personal care products, household cleaning products, aerosols, paints and plasticisers. Default values for exposure levels will be required when measured information is not available, and measured information will depend on scenario – thus the combination of algorithm and product use scenario is

Box 9.3 Algorithms for use with estimating consumer exposure.

Inhalation exposure

$$C_{air} = q.w_f.R.V_r^{-1} \qquad (mg\ m^{-3})$$

$$I_{inh1} = C_{air}.V_{inh}.t \qquad (mg\ event^{-1})$$

$$I_{inh2} = I_{inh1}.BW^{-1} \qquad (mg\ kg^{-1}\ BW\ event^{-1})$$

$$I_{inh3} = I_{inh2}.n \qquad (mg\ kg^{-1}\ BW\ day^{-1})$$

C_{air}, average concentration in air (mg m^{-3}); q, amount of product used (mg); w_f, weight fraction of substance in product; R, respirable or inhalable fraction of product (default = 1 or all of the product inhaled); V_r, room volume (m^3); V_{inh}, ventilation rate for adults (default 0.8 m^3 h^{-1} or 20 m^3 day^{-1}); t, duration of exposure (hours); I_{inh}, amount of substance inhaled/respired; BW, body weight (default adult values: female, 60 kg; male, 70 kg); n, number of events (per day).

Dermal exposure

$$C_{der} = d.w_f \qquad (mg\ cm^{-1})*$$

$$E_{der1} = C_{der}.T_{der}.S_{der} \qquad (mg\ event^{-1})$$

$$E_{der2} = E_{der1}.n.BW^{-1} \qquad (mg\ kg^{-1}\ BW\ day^{-1})$$

*of substance in product

C_{der}, average concentration in product (mg); d, density of product (mg m^{-3}); w_f, weight fraction of substance in product; E_{der}, amount of substance on skin; T_{der}, thickness of layer in product (cm); S_{der}, surface area of exposed skin (cm^2); n, number of events (per day); BW, body weight (kg).

Oral exposure

$$I_{orl} = q.w_f.f_{orl} \qquad (mg\ event^{-1})$$

I_{orl}, amount of substance ingested (mg); q, amount of product used (mg); w_f, weight fraction of substance in product; f_{orl}, fraction of product swallowed.

Note
From HSC (1994).

the exposure model. The results obtained from the model can then be set against NOAELs (or near equivalents) to obtain a margin of exposure. Two examples are given in Box 9.4. Monitoring in use or in simulation can be used to confirm the value of the model.

More specific procedures may apply to many substances when used as, for example, cosmetics, toys, food contact materials, biocides and pharmaceuticals.

Summary

The risk associated with intake and uptake standards is risk of end-effect being manifest at a particular dose (concentration and duration of exposure

Box 9.4 Two scenarios for consumer product exposure.

Hair spray
Weight of product used per event, 1000 mg; fraction of substance in product, 1 per cent (10 mg); inhalable fraction, 70 per cent; 'room volume', equivalent to 3 m³ (in the vicinity of use); volume inhaled, 0.8 m³ hour⁻¹ (default value); exposure time, 6 minutes (0.1 hour); bodyweight, 60 kg; product used three times per day.

$$C_{air} = \frac{1000 \times 0.01 \times 0.7}{3} = 23.3 \,mg\,m^{-3}$$

$$I_{inh1} = 23.3 \times 0.8 \times 0.1 = 1.86 \text{ mg event}^{-1}$$

$$I_{inh2} = 1.86/60 \qquad = 0.031 \text{ mg kg}^{-1} \text{ BW event}^{-1}$$

$$I_{inh3} = 0.031 \times 3 \qquad = 0.093 \text{ mg kg}^{-1} \text{ BW day}^{-1}$$

Dye from a T-shirt
Amount of dyestuff per cm² of fabric, 0.6 mg; weight fraction of substance in dyestuff, 30 per cent; fraction of dyestuff migrating from the T-shirt (first wearing), 0.001 per cent; surface area of exposed skin, 7500 cm².

$$E_{der} = 0.6 \times 0.3 \times 0.00001 \times 7500 = 0.0135 \text{ mg}$$

As this is for the first wearing period, there is no time factor attached to the value obtained.

Note
Both these examples use hypothetical values for the parameters entered into the equations given in Box 9.3.

to agent). Exposure information is used to determine the feasibility of the standard (exposure assessment) and to monitor the effectiveness of risk management.

The risk associated with input standards is the risk of placing a hazardous amount of agent in the medium (environment, food basket, etc.), i.e. of supplying sufficient material to the medium such that the input standard may be exceeded. There is an assessment of the source and the release pattern in order to derive an exposure assessment. The NOAEL, reference dose or standard is treated as the hazard and the attendant uncertainty is uncertainty associated with defining the hazard. Assumptions and models are used to translate from input into the intake (or vice versa). Monitoring data concerning inputs are also a part of risk management, ensuring that input standards are adhered to.

Chapter 10

The special case of major accident hazards

Major accident hazards are a special case. A 'major hazard' is defined as an imprecise term for a large-scale chemical hazard, especially one which may be released through an acute event (Jones, 1992). Thus, although major hazards include hazards from point sources, such as industrial plant and natural hazards such as emissions from volcano and lakes, they also include hazards from 'disseminated' sources such as those associated with food poisoning. Some examples of disasters, the manifestations of major accidents, are given in Table 10.1 and further examples are given in Illing (1999b). The toxicology associated with 'point source' major hazards is concerned with prediction and mitigation as well as the more conventional forms of prevention. It is aimed at providing ill-health information for predicting areas around a possible source (usually an industrial plant) likely to be affected by the effects of a single large dose of a chemical. It also includes the identification of potential methods of treatment in the event of an accident.

As the source of exposure is rarely easily identified in disseminated disasters, the toxicology associated with prevention of disseminated hazards must be that associated with maintenance of exposure sufficiently low that ill-health is prevented. This includes assessment using the process described previously (Chapters 7–9) and sufficiently rigorous enforcement to ensure that the standards and other management procedures developed as a result of the assessment are adhered to. Thus, managing the prevention of disseminated disasters is essentially similar to the management of covenanted releases from point sources – ensuring that exposure never reaches toxic levels. In addition, there will be a role associated with investigating incidents and tracing back from end-effect to source of exposure.

The remainder of this chapter is concerned with the prevention and mitigation role associated with point source major accident hazards. Usually, the source of the toxicant is more readily identifiable, and, like the risk assessments for 'input' standards, the risk assessments in this chapter are concerned with risk associated with the release of a hazardous quantity of an agent. It treats probability of end-effect for the dose (the usual 'risk' for a given dose) as part of the uncertainty in defining the hazard. Because the risk is associated with the identification of the source and size of release and the dispersion pattern for these releases, the risks can be tied to geographic area. Thus, both individual risk and societal risk (see Chapter 1) can be examined.

The regulatory scene for major hazards

Essentially, there are three circumstances associated with regulating toxic (or any other) major hazards. The first is land-use planning, the second is preparation of 'safety cases' and the third is implementation of an emergency plan following a serious accident. Land-use planning is concerned with where to locate major hazards and to what extent they should be segregated from other developments around a site by buffer zones. The buffer zones may be greater for some types of development, such as hospitals, and less for offices and other industrial premises than for housing. The 'safety case' includes assessment of the likelihood of the event occurring, the design and implementation of preventative measures to reduce the likelihood of the event occurring and 'on-site' and 'off-site' emergency planning. Figure 10.1 shows the routes by which toxic effects may become manifest.

The general approach to major hazards

The toxicology associated with major hazards is essentially predictive. It has to fit with the approaches used to describe the likelihood and size of release and the dispersion pattern for the toxicant. The overall process can be divided into seven steps:

- identification of possible hazardous release events;
- identification and analysis of the failure mechanisms which would allow such a release;
- estimation of rates and duration of releases;
- estimation of the frequencies of releases using the analysis of failure mechanisms;
- estimation of the injury consequences of the releases, taking account of mitigating factors;
- combination of the frequencies and consequences to determine the overall risk levels;
- judgement of the significance of the risk levels (by comparison with appropriate criteria).

The critical difference between risk assessment for major hazards and for other purposes is the need to predict frequency and size of potential accidental release. When dealing with covenanted releases, exposure is predicated and the aim is to decide on the maximum acceptable release.

A major hazards risk assessment can be described in three elements – a

Table 10.1 Some disasters involving toxic agents

Disaster	Cause	Effects
Seveso, Italy, 1976	Plant produced trichlorophenol from tetrachloro-benzene and sodium hydroxide. Solvent partially distilled off. At the end of the shift, heating and agitation switched off. About 7 hours later, a safety plate blew and the reaction mixture was vented to the atmosphere. Some 2–3 kg of Dioxin (2,3,7,8-tetrachlorodibenzo-p-dioxin) settled downwind of the plant.	Chloracne. Possible minor liver damage. Fear of cancer and reproductive effects not confirmed at 10 years after the event.
Toxic oil syndrome, Spain, 1981	Not fully understood. Mostly associated with oil denatured for industrial use being re-refined and sold for food use by itinerant salesmen.	Acute pleuropneumonia causing respiratory distress and death in severe cases, followed by a chronic phase, a sensorimotor peripheral neuropathy with sclerodermal-like skin changes. A total of 340 deaths and over 20,000 cases in approximately 2 years.
Bhopal, India, 1984	Release of methyl isocyanate from a factory manufacturing carbaryl. Introduction of water into a storage tank, resulted in production of carbon dioxide in a runaway exothermic reaction. The evolution of gas led to pressure build up; 30–35 tonnes vented over 2–3 hours at night. Plume dispersed over a densely populated area.	Estimates of deaths vary between 1,700 and 5,000, with up to 60,000 being seriously injured. Survivors reported that the vapour cloud gave off heat and had a pungent odour. Irritation, coughing and choking were followed by vomiting, defecation and urination, panic, depression, agitation, apathy and convulsions. Severe eye effects, including temporary blindness, did not persist. Initial lung effects (oedema, focal atelectasis) were probable causes of death and led, in survivors, to more persistent changes in lung function, and possible fibrosis and inflammation, which persisted in some cases.

Manchester Airport crash, 1985	British Airtours Boeing 737 bound for Corfu suffered uncontained failure in left engine which punctured fuel tank. Leaking fuel ignited. Pilot aborted take-off and turned onto taxiway and flames entered cabin through aft door. Airport fire service attended promptly, but could not prevent destruction of the aircraft.	Forty-seven passengers died immediately from inhalation of 'burning, painful' smoke; six from thermal injuries. There were thirty-eight survivors who reported drowsiness and disorientation, and one smoke death 6 days after the recovery as a result of severe pulmonary oedema and associated pneumonia.
Chernobyl, Ukraine, 1986	Core disintegration resulted in release of considerable quantities of radioactive material which was deposited over a wide geographic area of Ukraine and Belarus	Thirty-one immediate deaths from acute radiation sickness. Childhood thyroid cancer incidence elevated after 3 years, with a clear centring of the increase on the area surrounding Chernobyl. No increase seen outside the former USSR. Too early for observation of many other cancers.
Lake Nyos, Cameroon, 1986	Catastrophic release of gas (probably carbon dioxide) from a lake. Cloud was denser than air and dispersed through the river valley. It was lethal up to 10 km from the source.	About 1,700 human deaths and 3,000 animal deaths 6–36 hours after the event, probably due to carbon dioxide poisoning.
Tokyo subway, 1995	Sarin (an organophosphorous nerve agent) was released in a terrorist attack.	Ten people died; over 5,000 poisoned. Classic symptoms of organophosphate poisoning observed.

Note
From Illing (1999b).

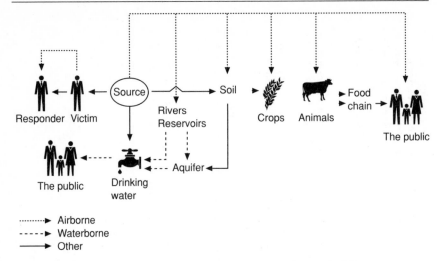

Figure 10.1 Potential pathways of human exposure to chemicals following a major accident. From IPCS (1999).

description of source, a model for looking at the dispersion of the substance, and a means of entering into the dispersion model parameters describing the conditions that will give a biological effect. Models have been developed for airborne dispersion, dispersion through ground and surface waters, soils and sediments, and dispersion through food chains.

The source term for inputting into the dispersion model may be obtained by 'fault tree' analysis of the frequency of events (failure rates), by 'event tree analysis' leading to an estimate of failure rates or by engineering judgements based on historical event frequency. The actual method(s) chosen will depend on the type of release being studied and the available data. The sizes and duration of the postulated/actual releases are also examined. For land-use planning, there is a continuum of event frequencies and sizes. Usually, sets of release sizes and duration are selected from a continuum and assigned appropriate frequencies. For emergency planning, the best choice is the 'severe but reasonably foreseeable' event as the appropriate basis on which to plan. This is a modification from the source release term for covenanted releases (discharges), where there is an assumption of a controlled (or, at least, controllable) pattern of release for use with the dispersion modelling.

Dispersion models for airborne releases usually take into account the buoyant density of the released cloud under different weather conditions and the frequencies of the different types of weather conditions at the release site. The models are combined with information on sizes and duration of release in order to develop isopleths (concentration–time contours for particular sets of conditions) and information on the geography and frequencies and types of weather conditions in order to develop risk contours (Figure 10.2).

Effects from airborne chemicals tend to be direct, and airborne dispersion tends to be rapid (hours and days) and to depend on weather conditions. Consequently, only very basic protective measures (e.g. instructions to 'stay indoors') can be given after the event. Indirect effects may also occur following deposition onto ground or into water.

Dispersion through soil, surface water or ground water tends to be slower than dispersion in air. Although any river-based surface water model depends on knowledge of the river system and the flows of water from the different contributors under various conditions, and hence is river system specific, dispersion through river systems can be modelled. Models are also available for dispersion through soil and ground water. In addition, there may be a

Development of isopleth envelope. (The information on dispersion is three-dimensional and includes vertical as well as horizontal directions. Plumes from a stack can rise or go to ground level, depending on weather conditions. The required isopleth envelope is two-dimensional and refers to near-ground conditions.)	Incorporation of meteorological information, such as wind speed, direction and frequency and buoyancy conditions (annual averages)

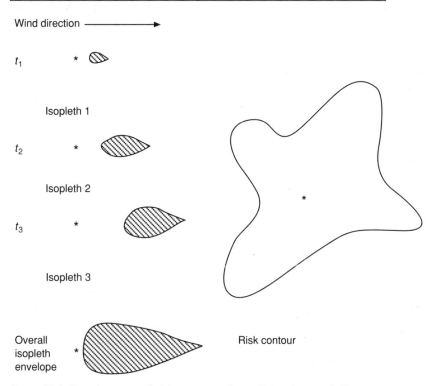

Figure 10.2 Development of risk contours from dispersion modelling.

need to examine the transfer between media – from air to water or soil to water – and fugacity models are available to deal with these situations (Mackay *et al.*, 1996a). There is a longer time period in which to take decisions concerning control of effects mediated through drinking water and food supplies than is normal for direct airborne dispersion, thus it is more likely that effective protective measures can be undertaken.

The toxicity associated with major hazards

The toxicity associated with airborne major hazards tends to be acute toxicity. Generally, it can be assumed that the release will be for a relatively short duration and exposure will be short term. This is a reasonable assumption as, if significant quantities of the toxicant are lodged in soil or water, steps will be taken to ensure that exposure through inhaling resuspended toxicant or from food and drinking water is kept suitably low. However, the levels of airborne exposure may well be such that death and serious ill-health requiring hospitalisation are potential consequences of these uncovenanted releases that have to be allowed for. This contrasts with covenanted discharges, where the emission or discharge limit is likely to be for discharges over a long period of time, steady-state concentrations may be generated and hence long-term exposure to the chemical needs examining. Levels of ill-health examined also differ as, for discharges, the dose–effect relationship and NOAEL or the dose–response relationship can be used to set a discharge limit at a level designed to ensure that the risk of any ill-health (severe or minor) is low. Essentially, major hazards toxicity is prediction of concentration–time (dose) thresholds that will cause various levels of ill-health rather than setting a maximum concentration–time combination (dose) which is unlikely to cause ill-health. Use of the uncertainty factor approach is therefore inappropriate.

The main method used for handling the toxicity is based on acute toxicity data (Illing, 1989; ECETOC, 1991; Fairhurst and Turner, 1993). There are some differences between land-use planning and safety case/emergency planning, so each will be considered separately.

Land-use planning criteria

Land-use planning can employ death as the harm criterion for human health effects, but sublethal effects may be serious and of great concern when handling toxicants. In consequence, the broader concept of the 'dangerous dose' has been used. It is defined as:

- severe distress will be caused to almost everyone;
- a substantial fraction will require medical attention;
- some people are seriously injured and require prolonged treatment;

- any highly susceptible people may be killed.

(Fairhurst and Turner, 1993)

An arbitrary ratio between the harm criterion for death and for a 'dangerous dose' has been elaborated by comparing the relationships for chlorine, ammonia, hydrogen fluoride and sulphur dioxide. The general relationship obtained is:

Dangerous dose = $LD_{50}/2.57$

(Franks *et al.*, 1996)

There also needs to be a harm criterion attached to this definition against which to judge the evidence concerning toxicity. The suggestion is that this represents a harm criterion of a likelihood of approximately one person in 10^6 (general population) receiving the dangerous dose per year (Health and Safety Executive, 1989). In addition, it was suggested that this corresponded to a 'harm criterion' of 3.3 people in 10^7 (general population) receiving a lethal dose, or of 3.3 people in 10^7 for a population with a high proportion of 'susceptible individuals' in it receiving a 'dangerous dose'. Homes for the elderly, caring institutions and long-stay hospitals are deemed to contain the high proportion of susceptible individuals. These values are convenient mathematically as they represent half an order of magnitude on a logarithmic scale. Obviously, these are general statements based on expert judgement and may require confirmation in individual cases once sufficient evidence becomes available.

Descriptive criteria are usually used for defining a major disaster to the environment in the UK (Department of the Environment, Transport and Regions, 2000). The criteria include definitions of different types of receptor and of thresholds of damage that apply. They were concerned with species and habitats, as well as damage to the built environment and damage to the environment that may lead to effects on human health (Table 10.2). These descriptions have not yet been linked to predictive information, thus any decision concerning the effects on the environment are based purely on expert judgements.

Emergency planning criteria

Emergency planning is essentially concerned with mitigating the consequences after an event has occurred. It involves both 'on-site' and 'off-site' planning and may cover immediate 'emergency' shutdown, responses of emergency services, the medical management of the immediate and longer term health effects, and the management of food and drinking water supplies and potential environmental effects (Murray, 1990; Home Office, 1994; Wells, 1997; IPCS, 1999; Chemical Incidents Response Service, 2000). The planning is concerned with a much wider range of biological effects than death. For

Table 10.2 UK Definitions of 'major accident to the environment'

Medium	Receptor	Threshold
Land/water (intertidal or near subtidal)	National nature reserves Sites of special scientific interest Marine nature reserves	>0.5 ha or >10% of the area adversely affected, whichever is the lesser >10% of an associated linear feature adversely affected >10% of a particular habitat or population of individual species adversely affected
Land/water	Natura 2000 or RAMSAR sites	>0.5 ha or 5% of the area of the site adversely affected >5% of an associated linear feature adversely affected >5% of a particular habitat or population of individual species adversely affected
Land	Other designated land: Environmentally sensitive areas Areas of outstanding national beauty Greenbelt land National parks Local nature reserves Wildlife Trust sites National Trust land Common land/country parks	>10% or 10 ha of land damaged, whichever is the lesser
Land/water	Scarce habitat: Biodiversity action plan habitats Geological features: caves, fossil beds, mineral veins, moraines, etc.	Damage to >10% of the area of the habitat or 2 ha, whichever is the lesser
Land/water	Widespread habitat: Habitat (including agricultural land) not otherwise classified	Contamination of 10 ha or more of land which for 1 year or more prevents the growing of crops, grazing of domestic animals or access to the public because of possible skin contact with dangerous substances or contamination of any aqueous habitat which prevents fishing or aquaculture or which similarly renders it inaccessible to the public
Water	Aquifers or groundwater	Any incident likely to require large-scale and long-term remedial measures or any incident of contamination/pollution by persistent compounds occurring within the most vulnerable groundwater resources (groundwater protection zone 1)

Land/water	Soil or sediment (to a depth of 1 metre)	Contamination or pollution of the receptor such that. Soil would be regarded as contaminated land (planned present or future uses could be compromised) Sediment would become loaded with sufficient material to compromise the chemical or biological quality of the overlying waters for any period in excess of a few days Deterioration of the biological quality of soil or sediment such that common organisms of these ecosystems were absent, the structure of the biological community altered for periods in excess of a season, or normal ecosystem function was severely impaired for a period in excess of 1 year
Land	Built heritage: Buildings Listed buildings	Damage to a Grade I (England and Wales) or category A (Scotland) or a scheduled ancient monument such that it no longer possesses its architectural, historic or archaeological importance, and which would result in it being de-listed or de-scheduled if no remedial/restorative work was undertaken or Damage to an area of archaeological importance or a conservation area similarly resulting in loss of importance
Water	Groundwater Drinking water Fish and shellfish water Bathing waters	Specific levels of exceedance of standards for continuous emissions standards should be considered in the post-remediation and restoration works
Land/air/water	Particular species: 'Common' species Species listed in European legislation Species listed in 'red data book'	Common species: where there are reliable estimates of species numbers, death of or serious sublethal effects within 1% of any species would be significant For common plant species, death of or serious sublethal effects within 5% of the ground cover For species of high value or with special protection the threshold may be lower than 1% or 5% and liaison with the appropriate statutory conservation organisation should be used to determine an appropriate threshold Where reliable estimates of population numbers do not exist, liaison with the statutory authority will be necessary to determine appropriate thresholds Any loss of a 'red data book' species or species site would be considered a major accident

Information from Department of the Environment, Transport and Regions (2000)

immediate effects on human health, these include 'severe health effects' (disability, requiring hospital treatment) and 'mild health effects' (discomfort or distress, detection or nuisance). Similar guidelines have been developed by a number of bodies. Those of ECETOC are given in Box 10.1 and a comparison of ECETOC's Emergency Exposure Limits and the US Acute Exposure Guidline Levels and Emergency Response Planning Guidelines is presented in Table 10.3. These definitions are essentially harm criteria for airborne concentrations for exposures lasting up to a specified time. These are criteria below which direct toxic effects are unlikely to lead to one of death/permanent incapacity, disability or discomfort. Although hospital treatment may be essential for recovery from severe health effects, it will usually have little influence in the case of milder effects (discomfort). The planning may also consider possible longer term exposure, protection of food and water supplies and possibly (if practicable) protection of the environment.

Fitting the toxicity information to the criteria

Usually, only acute toxicity data are available. The rare occasions where there is human experience concerning death and severe disablement are mainly when information on exposure is poor (warfare/terrorist attack/major accident experience), thus the data are usually obtained from animal studies.

Box 10.1 Definitions of emergency exposure indices.

Emergency exposure index 1
That airborne concentration for exposure lasting up to a specified time (t_1) <u>below</u> <u>which</u> direct toxic effects are unlikely to lead to *discomfort* in the exposed population (including susceptible, but excluding hypersusceptible, groups), and <u>above</u> <u>which</u>, as the concentration increases, discomfort would become increasingly more common.

Emergency exposure index 2
That airborne concentration for exposures lasting up to a specified time (t_2) <u>below</u> <u>which</u> direct toxic effects are unlikely to lead to *disability* (the need for rescue and treatment) in the exposed population (including susceptible, but excluding hypersusceptible, groups), and <u>above</u> <u>which</u>, as the concentration increases, disability would become increasingly more common.

Emergency exposure index 3
That airborne concentration for exposures lasting up to a specified time (t_3) <u>below</u> <u>which</u> direct toxic effects are unlikely to lead to *death/permanent incapacity* in the exposed population (including susceptible, but excluding hypersusceptible, groups) and above which, as the concentration increases, death or permanent incapacity becomes increasingly common.

Note
From ECETOC (1991).

Table 10.3 Relationship between Emergency Exposure Limits (EELs), Acute Exposure Guideline Levels (AEGLs) and Emergency Response Planning Guidelines (ERPGs).

	EEl	AEGL	ERPG
Source of definition	European Chemical Industry Ecotoxicology and Toxicology Centre	US National Advisory Committee	American Industrial Hygiene Association
Time frame	Definition requires that time is stated, but does not specify the time	0.5, 1, 4 or 8 h	1 h

From ECETOC (1991) and IPCS (1999).

It is much more likely that occupational health experience will be able to assist when dealing with discomfort or nuisance, where there is likely to be human experience. As most exposure is likely to be by inhalation, inhalation studies are the preferred studies for assessing major hazard acute toxicity. If whole body studies are conducted, then there is no need to allow separately for skin absorption.

The data from the most sensitive relevant species are selected to represent human responsiveness. Generally, a concentration–time relationship is needed. Thus, the LCT_{50} or ECT_{50} [concentration–time relationship resulting in 50 per cent mortality (L) or effect (E)] is derived. In the early years of the twentieth century, when examining lethality, the relationship:

$$ct = \text{constant}$$

where c is concentration and t is time was obtained, and it subsequently became known as the Haber rule. More recent observations suggest the general relationship is:

$$c^n t = \text{constant}$$

Although a wide range of values for n has been cited, usually the value appears to be close to 1 or to 2. In the absence of further information, a default value of 1 is commonly used.

Normally, the 50 per cent values (the LCT_{50} or ECT_{50}) are transformed to another set of values to represent a low percentage (1–5 per cent) of deaths or effects. Probit analysis, using 'best estimate' data for a single strain and species, may be used to carry out this transformation if direct observation is difficult. If a concentration–time relationship has been derived from modern studies based on the 'fixed dose' procedure and 'evident toxicity', the set of

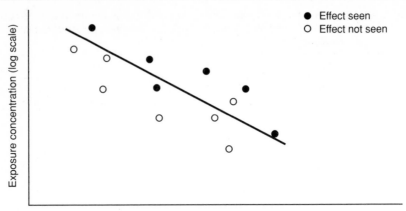

Figure 10.3 Idealised scatter diagram to determine the boundary conditions of an exposure–time relationship for lethality. By plotting on logarithmic axes, the slope of the boundary line can be used to derive *n*. A slope of –2 indicates that the value for *n* in the equation $c^n t$ = constant is 2.

values representing a low percentage of deaths would be obtained directly. However, most of the relevant substances have been well-known toxicants for a long time, so this is unlikely to be the case. Toxicological judgement is applied to allow for heterogeneity in the human population. The assessment of phosgene toxicity by the Major Hazards Assessment Panel working party (MHAP, 1993) is an example of the use of this technique.

Other approaches to the relevant acute toxicological evaluation include a boundary condition approach (ECETOC, 1991; Figure 10.3) and a categorisation scheme (Bridges, 1990).

Other data, if available, are assessed qualitatively.

Conclusion

The area of major hazards toxicity is still developing. The field has been dominated by the psychometric paradigm for risk analysis and engineering approaches to predicting likelihood, size and duration of exposure. The contribution of toxicologists and ecotoxicologists to this type of risk assessment has been limited, possibly because of the need for a non-traditional approach to toxicological/ecotoxicological risk assessment. For human health effects, problems arise from the use of numerical values for 'best estimate' rather than 'conservative' predictions. For effects on the environment, criteria and thresholds for harm have been defined. However, these criteria do not relate directly to the results of predictive testing, hence it is difficult to relate parameters of concentration and duration of chemical exposure to them. These problems might have been exacerbated by difficulties of communication between numerate (engineering based) and literate (biologically based) risk assessors.

Chapter 11

Evaluation of effects on the environment

Effects on the environment include effects on the built environment as well as effects on the natural environment. Although effects on ecosystems involving humans can be considered as part of effects on the environment, wider effects and effects on ecosystems not involving humans are the main effects of interest in this chapter. Areas usually covered are given in Box 11.1.

In contrast to the situation for human health, where risk to the individual is usually the first concern, when dealing with non-human health environmental effects the risk to the population is normally the more important. In principle, both input and intake standards can be set. Usually, the management of the risk is by control of input or by remediation, and the risk being examined is that associated with an initiating event (release of the agent), with uncertainties in the relationship between intake (by the organism or the ecosystem) and end-effect as part of the uncertainty in defining the hazard.

In this chapter we will cover the whole of the risk characterisation, including hazard identification and characterisation and exposure assessment. As the process described is used to derive a ratio, risk evaluation (determining whether the ratio of hazard to exposure is satisfactory) is carried out separately as the first stage of the risk management.

The approach to identifying effects on human health described in Chapter 8 is applicable to the identification of effects in any individual species, although the test species will be chosen as an index for the relevant non-human species rather than as an index for humans. However, ecotoxicology is concerned with more than just the individual species, it is also the natural extension of toxicology concerned with populations, food webs and ecosystems. The ecological significance of a toxic effect, or lack of it, may be indirect. A clear example of an indirect effect would be the loss of a species due to deliberate poisoning (and hence elimination) of its food supply, a problem often associated with the use of pesticides in agriculture.

Box 11.1 Areas of ecotoxicity that should be covered in a risk assessment.

Aquatic environment
Short-term, long-term and reproductive toxicity in algae (primary producer), arthropods (*Daphnia*, primary consumer) and fish (tertiary consumer). These include laboratory studies and studies in micro- and mesocosms.

Terrestrial environment
Tests should cover:

- Primary production (plants)
- Decomposing capacity of soil (litter consumers/microorganisms)
- Invertebrate soil fauna (herbivores, fungivores, saprovores)
- Studies on honey bees
- Vertebrates (omnivores/carnivores)

These include laboratory studies, studies in micro- and mesocosms and field trials.

Note
Based on Health and Safety Executive (1994).

Ecosystem, community, trophic level and food chain/web

Before dealing with ecotoxicology, some ecological concepts must be defined. Ecology is a complex biological discipline, with its own terminology and concepts. Key elements to keep in mind when considering ecotoxicological risk assessment are the ecosystem, the community, the trophic level and the food chain/web. The definitions given here are from Begon *et al.* (1990).

An ecosystem is 'a holistic concept of the plants, the animals habitually associated with them and all the physical and chemical components of their immediate environment or habitat which together form a recognisable, self-contained entity'. An ecological community is the reality on the ground, the species that occur together in space and time. Agro-ecosystems are ecosystems deliberately manipulated in order to grow plants for human consumption. Plant protection products and biocides are chemicals that are deliberately applied to specific communities to cause certain effects on those communities. They can spill over into (and damage) other communities. Exposure to other chemicals is usually incidental or accidental, although there will be communities adapted to accommodating chemicals, etc. associated with sewage and waste disposal that can be considered as ecosystems.

A trophic level is 'a position in a food chain assessed by the number of energy transfer steps to reach that level'. A food chain is an abstract representation of the links between consumer and consumed populations (Table 11.1). In practice, a consumer species rarely exists on a single source of food, and may take food species from several trophic levels within a food

Table 11.1 Examples of food chains

	Trophic level	Food chain 1	Food chain 2	Food chain 3
Primary producer	1	Algae	Pine trees	Grasses
Secondary producer (primary consumer)	2	*Daphnia*	Aphids	Farm animals
Secondary consumer	3	Water spider	Spiders	
Tertiary consumer	4	Fish	Tits and warblers (birds)	
Quaternary consumer (top predator)	5	Pike, birds of prey	Birds of prey (hawks)	Humans

Note
These are examples of three possible food chains among many, including the chain associated with clearing dead organic matter (by detritovores). The primary producer is an autotroph; the remainder are heterotrophs. The third chain is that of the agro-ecosystem, and illustrates that different chains may contain different numbers of trophic levels. In addition, it is quite possible for a species to occupy more than one trophic level within a chain.

chain. A more realistic way of setting out the food supply has to account for the several sources of food that may arise from different trophic levels. A food web is a more complex attempt to describe the feeding relationships in a community that includes all the links revealed by dietary analysis (Figure 11.1).

Bioconcentration of chemicals to toxic levels may occur in an individual species within a food chain. Biomagnification may occur through several of the trophic levels such that toxic effects occur in the 'top predator' [birds such as eagles, hawks, ospreys and owls, fish-eating fish such as pike (*Esox lucius*)] and carnivorous mammals such as fox and cat may be poisoned secondarily. Dichloro-diphenyl-trichloroethane (DDT) caused eggshell thinning in birds of prey (raptors), and hence sharp decreases in the populations of these top predators, as a result of bioconcentration and biomagnification through the food web.

Another possible ecotoxic effect includes removal of one or several elements in a trophic level, with consequent loss of food supplies for the members of higher trophic levels in the community, and hence decrease in their population size. Losses of insectivorous birds in an agricultural environment could be accounted for, at least in part, by removal of their food supply through enthusiastic application of broad-spectrum pesticides.

As this book is aimed at discussing risk assessment, these ecological concepts will not be further discussed here. Further information on ecology and ecotoxicology can be obtained from any appropriate text.

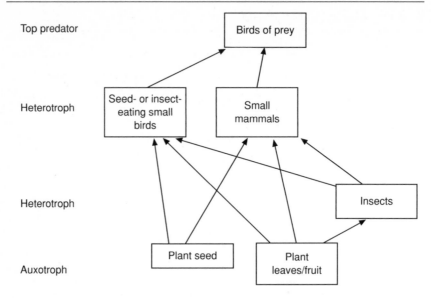

Figure 11.1 A simplified example of a food web. This generalised food web is one associated with the passage of organochlorines used as insecticides. The organochlorines were concentrated through the food web and caused eggshell thinning in the top predators, the birds of prey. The populations of the birds of prey in affected areas were severely reduced as a consequence of breeding failures due to the eggshell thinning. Organochlorine pesticides are, in the main, no longer considered acceptable.

Toxicity–exposure ratio (TER), predicted exposure concentration (PEC) and predicted no-effect concentration (PNEC)

The first approach to environmental risk assessment for a substance not already present is to consider direct toxicity to a given species. Either the 'toxicity–exposure ratio' (TER) or the inverse of the TER, usually known as the PEC/PNEC ratio, can be used to describe that toxicity. The TER is derived from a toxicological parameter such as the LC_{50} or the 'predicted no-effect concentration' (PNEC; derived from toxicological information such as the no observed effect concentration) and 'predicted exposure concentration' (PEC; derived from measured or modelled information):

$$TER = \frac{PNEC \left(\text{or other biological parameter}\right)}{PEC}$$

The TER is essentially a risk estimate analogous to the 'margin of exposure' employed in human health toxicology. It includes the hazard identification, hazard evaluation, exposure assessment and risk characterisation stages of risk assessment. The larger the value the less the concern is for the risk. When the equation is inverted to obtain PEC/PNEC ratios, PEC/PNEC values of greater than 1 should lead to concern over the risks of environmental pollution. When there is concern arising from these ratios, some form of further testing or risk management should be considered, either immediately or at some later date, dependent on the amounts being placed in the environment and the effects seen. If that concern is sufficiently serious, the 'precautionary principle' should be applied and risk management undertaken at the same time as the assessment is being refined.

Both TER and PEC/PNEC are fairly crude approaches that can start with basic 'worst case' data and be refined, either by obtaining more sophisticated data or by altering the assumptions incorporated into the assessments. PNEC is derived from toxicity or ecotoxicity data. PEC is derived from information on fate and behaviour in the environmental medium, and may be for soil, ground or surface water or air. PEC therefore depends on information concerning the size of release and the way in which the release is dispersed into the environment. PEC may be for initial or longer term effects and may be local or regional in its applicability.

Types of data available

In the first stages of a risk assessment, the data required are usually relatively simple. They include physicochemical data and some acute toxicity data in potential indicator species. In due course, much more sophisticated data may be acquired, including data for individual species and data derived from experimental ecosystems (microcosms, mesocosms) and field studies. Essentially, exposure is assessed in studies on release and on fate and behaviour, and in studies examining bioaccumulation and biomagnification; hazard is assessed in studies on toxicity in indicator species.

Release/discharge

Prediction of environmental concentrations depends on knowledge of what, where, when and how any release or discharge occurs. It also depends on any treatment undertaken during the release process. Release may occur at any stage in the life cycle of a product (Table 11.2).

How much is released or discharged and to what extent it can be controlled is important. If a product is a chemical intermediate, it may only ever be contained in a closed system and very little, if any, is ever released. In addition, a chemical may be released as a 'point source' release (from a factory) or widely dispersed, as commonly happens with plant protection products or detergents.

Table 11.2 Factors affecting emissions of substances to the environment.

'Life' of the chemical	Waste treatment	Environment
Production	Minimise and recycle	Air
Formulation (blending, mixing to make preparations)	Waste water treatment plant	Surface and ground water (and sediment)
Use Industry (large-scale professional)	Waste gases treatment (e.g. flue desulphurisation)	Soil Biota (organisms)
Trade (small-scale professional) Individual consumer (personal)	Incineration	
Disposal (including waste treatment)		

Fate and behaviour

Air, soil, surface and ground water are all media for which predicted environmental concentrations may be required. Waste arising from production, formulation, storage and use may be discharged directly to an environmental compartment or treated before its appearance in the environment (Table 11.2). In order to keep damage to the environment to a minimum, emphasis is being placed on minimising the amounts of waste produced and waste recycling. In addition, chemical pollutants in wastes may be treated prior to their appearance in the environment, and this must be allowed for in determining the PEC. Treatment of wastewater containing pollutants prior to discharge to the aqueous environment is a particular example.

Wastewater treatment

A chemical can be removed during wastewater treatment in sewage treatment works. In effect, sewage treatment occurs in four stages. These are:

1   preliminary treatment to remove or macerate material likely to cause blockages and to allow inorganic grit to settle out;
2   primary settlement to allow most of the solid particles to settle by gravity;
3   secondary treatment is a biological treatment stage where, normally, microorganisms oxidise the settled sewage (anaerobic degradation is sometimes used);
4   tertiary treatment which may include removal of residual solids, ammonia, nitrate and phosphorus and/or disinfection.

Often, sewage treatment works only undertake one or two of the outlined stages. The output from the sewage treatment works will be relatively purer water and sludge that may contain relatively large amounts of pollutants. A diagrammatic representation of the full process is given in Figure 11.2.

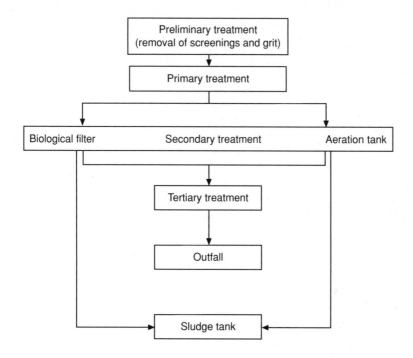

Primary treatment	Secondary treatment	Tertiary treatment
Solids separated out by gravity Primary sludge drawn off for treatment and disposal	Biological treatment Requires a reactor and a secondary sedimentation tank. Aerobic process (percolating filter bed containing suitable microorganisms or aeration tank containing activated sludge)	Not usually undertaken, but may include removal of solids, ammonia, nitrate and/or phosphorus. May also include disinfecting
Sludge may be spread on farmland or disposed of to landfill. Anaerobic digestion may be undertaken to render the sludge relatively inoffensive, and the methane produced can be used to produce heat		

Figure 11.2 Sewage treatment. Further information can be obtained from Try and Price (1995).

Chemical pollutants may be degraded during treatment or they can, if present in too high a concentration, destroy the ability of the microbes present during secondary treatment to function. The degree of removal (P) of a pollutant from the wastewater is determined by the physicochemical properties of the substance (biodegradation, adsorption onto sludge, sedimentation of insoluble material and volatility). Early information can be obtained from laboratory data and modelling. Laboratory studies examining these interactions include octanol–water partition, 'ready biodegradation' tests and information based on Henry's law. If a substance is not readily biodegradable, then it may be tested for inherent biodegradability and/or in tests aimed at simulation of specific treatments. These data can be inputted into tables to determine the value of P.

When combined with information on dilution, it is possible to obtain an initial aqueous environmental PEC from the above data. Dilution depends on the volume of the receiving water. Instantaneous mixing is assumed. As most treatment plants discharge wastewater (after treatment) to flowing water (rivers), dilution depends on the flow rates of the water, and thus may depend on season. The PEC is obtained from the equation:

$$PEC_{initial} = W.Q^{-1}.(100 - P).D^{-1}.10^{-2}$$

where W is emission rate for the chemical (kg day^{-1}); Q is volume of waste water (m^3 day^{-1}) (estimated if necessary); P is degree of removal in the treatment works (per cent), obtained from tables; and D is the dilution factor for the water flow of the receiving river.

Other degradation processes may also need examination. These may include anaerobic degradation or biodegradation in sea water.

Pollutant may be retained on sludge, or metabolised by the microorganisms present, and the more volatile chemicals may be discharged to the air. Models can also be used to examine these discharges.

Environmental factors

Initial discharges to the environment are usually to water or air. Some airborne discharges (e.g. pesticide sprays) may rapidly fall to ground. Also, some discharge from point sources may be to landfill waste disposal sites, essentially large-scale bioreactors where pollutants may be degraded and/or slowly discharged to the more general environment through dispersion. Once in the environment, the chemical can interact with the components of the environment or transfer between environmental compartments.

Measurements used to examine abiotic removal processes include the potential for volatilisation from sludge, soil or water to air and the potential for adsorption/desorption on soil particles or sediment (Box 11.2). If a chemical has a high octanol–water partition coefficient, it is likely to be

Box 11.2 Calculation constants associated with mobility between media

---

Soil water distribution coefficient:

$$K_d = \frac{\left[\text{Chemical in aqueous phase}\right]}{\left[\left(\text{Total chemical}\right) - \left(\text{Chemical in aqueous phase}\right)\right]}$$

K_d is determined by mixing soil, water and the test chemical together and measuring the concentration of chemical in the aqueous phase. Values of < 2 indicate that the chemical is likely to be mobile.

Binding to organic material:

$$K_{oc} = \frac{K_d}{\% \text{ of organic carbon in sample}}$$

The organic carbon content of the soil sample is determined from the loss in weight when a dried soil sample is subjected to high-temperature combustion. Mobile chemicals have $K_{oc} < 500$.

Henry's law constant:

$$K_h = \frac{\left[\text{Test chemical in water}\right]}{\left[\text{Test chemical in water}\right]}$$

Mobile chemicals tend to have a constant $< 10^{-2}$ atm m^3 mol^{-1}.

Note
For further information, see Shaw and Chadwick (1998).

better adsorbed. Mobile chemicals likely to leach from soil to water tend to be water soluble and poor at binding to the organic material (e.g. humus) in soil. The Henry's law constant is of value when considering transfer from water to air.

Fugacity models, such as those described by Mackay *et al.* (1992, 1996a,b) can be used to describe the fate of a chemical in the environment at a regional (1,000,000 km^2) level. In the Mackay model, there are three levels of evaluation. The fate information obtained at each level is shown in Table 11.3. The level 1 model (the simplest) is a straightforward equilibrium model (Figure 11.3), based on steady-state conditions for partition among six media (air, water, soil, sediment, suspended sediment and fish). It makes assumptions concerning the volumes of each of these media. The level 2 model (Figure 11.4) also allows for inputs (emissions into the environment) and losses due to transport and degradation (at steady state). The level 3 model (Figure 11.5) does not assume equilibrium among the different media. It requires the development of intermedia transport rates for the various diffusive and non-diffusive processes involved in transport among media. It is data demanding and complex.

Table 11.3 The information obtainable from fugacity models

Model level	Conditions evaluated	Fate information obtained
Level 1	Equilibrium partition under steady state	The primary compartments to which the substance will partition and the approximate relative concentrations in the compartments, including tendency to bioaccumulate
Level 2	Includes losses by advective transport and degrading reactions	The approximate residence time or persistence in the environment, dominant mechanisms of loss by reaction and advection, or tendency for transport out of the generic environment in either air or water
Level 3	Non-equilibrium because includes intermedia transport processes, steady state	How fate is affected by medium of discharge, which intermedia transport processes are most important, and which processes account for contamination in media other than that receiving the discharge; persistence

Note
For further information, see Mackay *et al.* (1996b).

On the smaller scale, models of dispersion in air, in soil and ground water, or in river and coastal waters may be required. Many of these are essentially those described in Chapters 9 and 10, so they will not be repeated here. The principal difference will be that the concentration–time relationship for harm will be for an ecotoxicological effect, rather than for an effect on human health.

Toxicity in indicator species

Clearly, it is not possible to test every chemical likely to be placed in the environment in all species likely to be found in a particular environment. Reducing the amount of testing to reasonable levels involves the use of indicator species. In addition to acute toxicity to adults, testing can include that for effects on prolonged exposure and tests for effects on reproduction and on early life stages of indicator organisms. A selection of indicator species is given in Box 11.3. Some of the indicator species have been chosen because of ease of handling in the laboratory environment and because the target species (e.g. birds of prey) are endangered species, consequently they are not member species for the trophic level of the target species. Nevertheless, their handling of the pollutant is considered similar enough for them to be satisfactory indicators. The parameters obtained from these toxicity tests vary according to the test. For algae, the concentration inhibiting the growth

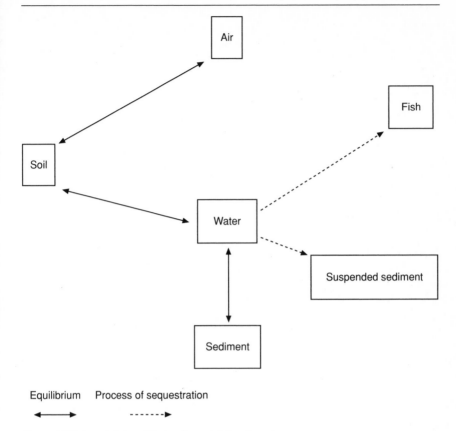

Figure 11.3 Level I (equilibrium) model for fugacity.

by 50 per cent is the usual parameter. For animals, the LC_{50}, the concentration causing 50 per cent of the animals to die, is used for acute toxicity and the no observed adverse effect concentration is the data point obtained from studies on the longer term and reproductive effects. In higher plants, the concentration just causing an effect is preferred.

Bioaccumulation, bioconcentration and biomagnification

Bioaccumulation and bioconcentration are related to direct uptake; biomagnification is related to uptake via the food chain through different pathways and involving different trophic levels. Bioaccumulation is usually measured using the octanol–water partition coefficient, determined experimentally or obtained by calculation. Values of log P (the logarithm to the base 10 of the coefficient) greater than three (and less than 6) indicates a potential for bioaccumulation. Within certain limitations, the biological

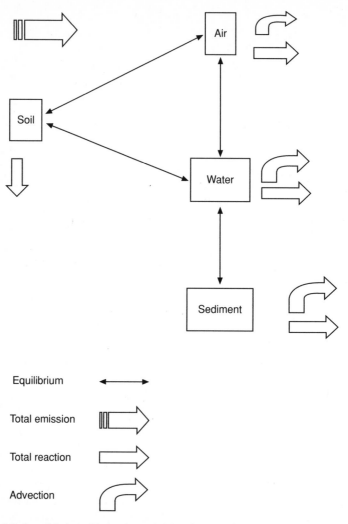

Figure 11.4 Level 2 (equilibrium) model for fugacity. The suspended sediment and fish elements have not been segregated from the water compartment.

concentration factor (BCF) correlates the log P. These limitations include the presence of active transport phenomena, metabolism and accumulation of metabolites, and tissue interactions. Biomagnification can lead to secondary poisoning. This requires a combination of the PEC in the relevant medium and the BCF to derive the concentration in the food species, and comparison with the predicted no-effect concentration (PNEC) in food, usually derived from studies on the relevant indicator species for the predator, usually a bird or mammal. If there is passage through several trophic levels,

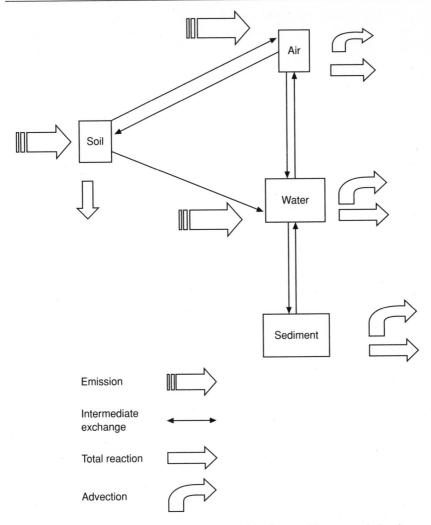

Figure 11.5 Level 3 (intermedia transport) model for fugacity. The suspended sediment and fish elements have not been segregated from the water compartment.

the calculation will need to be repeated several times in order to develop conclusions concerning the top predator.

Removal of a trophic level

Generally, pesticides are aimed at removing or minimising damage from species considered harmful to the crop being produced. However, pesticides are rarely sufficiently specific that they only kill the species causing the damage, they also affect other neutral or beneficial organisms (collateral

Box 11.3 Test species for environmental toxicity.

Algae (freshwater aquatic)
Biomass production for:
   Selenastrum capricornutum
   Scenedescemus subspicatus
   Chlorella vulgaris

Higher plants (terrestrial)
Growth can be studied in many species. Germination frequency, root elongation and shoot elongation are measured. The OECD has divided species into three groups, and suggests testing in one species from each group.

Group 1:	(Monocotyledons)
	Lolium perenne (ryegrass)
	Oryza sativa (rice)
	Avena sativa (oats)
	Triticum aestivum (wheat)
	Sorghum bicolor (sorghum)
Group 2:	(Brassicas)
	Brassica alba (mustard)
	Brassica napus (oil seed rape/canola)
	Raphanus sativus (radish)
	Brassica rapa (turnip)
	Brassica campestris var. chinesiensis (Chinese cabbage)
Group 3:	(Legumes, etc.)
	Vicia sativa (vetch)
	Phaseolus aureus (mung bean)
	Trifolium praetense (red clover)
	Trifolium ornitopodioides (fenugreek)
	Lactuta sativa (lettuce)
	Lepidium sativum (cress)

Earthworm (terrestrial)
   Eisenia foetida

Arthropods
   Daphnia magna (fresh water aquatic primary consumer)
   [*Artemia salina* (brine shrimp) may be used if a salt-water species is required]
   Caribid beetles (spring breeders and/or autumn breeders) (beneficial terrestrial–soil)
   Staphylinid beetles (beneficial terrestrial–soil)
   Spiders (*Linyphidae, Lycosidae*) (beneficial terrestrial–soil)
   Aphids (beneficial terrestrial–soil)
   Sawfly larvae, Heteropters, small caribids, Chrysomelidae, Curculionidae (food insects for game bird chicks)
   Apis mellifera (honey bee) (terrestrial–airborne pollinator)

Fish (aqueous)
Acute/chronic toxicity
   Brachydanio rerio (zebrafish)* – warm flowing freshwater
   Pimephales promelas (fathead minnow)* – estuarine

Cyprianus carpio (common carp) – still cold freshwater
Oryzias latipes (ricefish)*
Poecilia reticulata (Guppy) – warm still freshwater
Lepomis macrochirus (bluegill) – cold still or flowing freshwater
Oncorhynchus mykiss (rainbow trout)* – flowing cold freshwater
*These species are considered suitable for studying early life effects; *Cyprionodon variegatus* (sheepshead minnow) is a saltwater species also considered suitable for conducting studies on early life effects. Although not considered for the purposes of toxicity testing, fish can also be divided into benthic (bottom-feeders) or pelagic.

Birds
Species for toxicity testing
  Alectoris rufa (red-legged partridge)
  Anas platyrhynchos (mallard)†
  Colinus virginianus (bobwhite quail)†
  Columbia livia (pigeon)
  Coturnix c. japonica (Japanese quail)†
  Phasianus colchicus (ring-necked pheasant)
†Avian reproduction can be studied in these species. Although none of these species is a top predator, they are used to represent the raptors as most raptors are predators.

Mammals (mainly terrestrial)
Normally, the index species and end-points used for mammalian toxicity are the same as those used for studying human health effects, namely acute, repeated dose, reproduction, etc. toxicity in rat, mouse, rabbit, marmoset, dog and various monkey species.
  [It has been suggested (Shaw and Chadwick, 1998) that trophic level 2 is represented by *Daphnia* and *Artemia*; trophic level 3 by other arthropods; trophic level 4 by the fish tests; and trophic level 5 by the bird tests. Clearly, this is simplistic and takes no account of the information available from mammalian testing.]

Note
From OECD (1981), HSE/MAFF (date not stated) and Shaw and Chadwick (1998).

damage). This lack of specificity means that, with pesticides, it is possible to cause indirect effects on the populations of organisms at higher trophic levels in a community by removal of their food supplies.

Monitoring

Exposure monitoring can be used to confirm the validity of the determination of the PEC, and hence to modify the risk assessment, once exposure takes place. Surveys of wildlife data can be used to monitor effects. Field trials are used to confirm that the ecotoxicological risk assessments derived from laboratory and microcosm/mesocosm studies are satisfactory, and to cover areas of ecotoxicology not readily testable in laboratory conditions. Wildlife incident appraisal schemes and time series of wildlife surveys can check that, in real life practice, the assessments are valid and/or identify problems.

Conclusion

Most ecotoxicological risk assessment is judgemental in character, and is concerned with populations and species. It starts with very basic predictive information that can be refined if the assessment shows this to be necessary. The biological processes being investigated are inherently complex and the predictive information is obtained from grossly simplified models and experimental systems. In addition, the relationships among experimental data, effects in the field and the criteria used to judge the adequacy of the TER or PEC/PNEC ratios are often ill defined. Although quantitative approaches may be employed in developing the information used in the risk assessment, the currently available data and risk assessment procedures are not suitable for use in numerical, quantitative risk assessment. Judgmental approaches, backed up by monitoring data, are likely to remain with us for the foreseeable future, and only in the most complex cases will it be worthwhile to develop the information and models for quantitative numerical risk assessment.

Chapter 12

Effects on the atmosphere

When dealing with effects on the atmosphere, the risk management is concerned with inputs into the atmosphere. The risks are therefore risks associated with the release of the agent, and uncertainties concerning the relationship between amount in the atmosphere and end-effect are uncertainties in defining the hazard. It is more difficult to disentangle effects on human health and effects on the wider environment. Although we may be dealing with regional or global effects, many atmospheric pollutants cross national boundaries. Control of much atmospheric pollution is based on international agreements. To an extent, transnational effects also occur when dealing with the aqueous environment, as with some of the major river systems and the North Sea, and are dealt with on the basis of international agreements, such as the 'OSPAR' (Oslo/Paris) agreements concerning control of pollution of the North Sea. However, international agreements become a much more notable feature of risk assessment when dealing with transnational air pollution problems and are the only effective ways by which global pollution problems can be tackled.

The structure of the atmosphere

The atmosphere can be considered as a series of spheres surrounding the earth (Figure 12.1). The troposphere is the part of the atmosphere lying immediately above the earth's surface, and can be divided into the boundary layer and the free troposphere. The boundary layer is bounded at its upper extreme by a temperature inversion. The stratosphere is the layer above the troposphere. At the interfaces between the different 'spheres' are a series of 'pauses'. There is a general circulation of air within the atmosphere, consequent on the input of solar energy and the rotation of the earth. That circulation includes a horizontal component, the general 'trade winds' and 'doldrums' known to mariners from the days of sailing vessels. It also includes a vertical component, composed in each hemisphere of three cells with an intertropical convergence zone at the equator and another mixing zone at each of the poles.

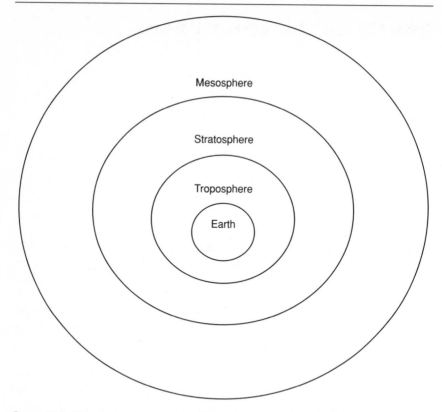

Figure 12.1 The atmosphere surrounding the earth and its layers. The boundaries are known as pauses; thus, the tropopause lies between the troposphere and the stratosphere, and the stratopause between the stratosphere and mesosphere. The mesopause marks the boundary with outer space.

There is also a cycle describing the behaviour of pollutants in the atmosphere. Emissions, which may be from man-made or natural sources, are transported or diffuse through the air and may be deposited dry or wet, unchanged or transformed, depending on weather conditions (Figure 12.2).

Effects on the atmosphere and their consequences

Chemicals may adversely affect the atmosphere in several ways (Box 12.1). These include local effects in the workplace or home, or urban air, regional effects over a wider geographic range (transnational pollution) and global effects affecting the world as a whole.

If a chemical is to be an atmospheric pollutant, it is usually a gas or a volatile liquid or easily sublimed solid, or it is deposited on particulate matter held suspended in air. The second parameter of importance will be its lifetime in the atmosphere.

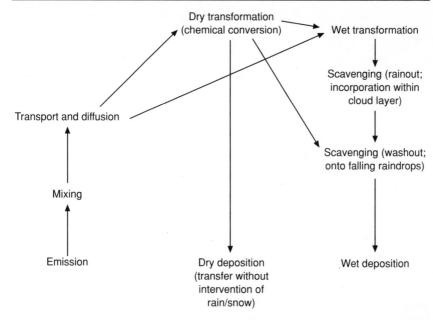

Figure 12.2 Atmospheric cycling processes for pollutants. Based on Harrison (1990).

In urban air, the primary pollutants are carbon dioxide, carbon monoxide, nitrogen oxides, sulphur dioxide and particles from hydrocarbon combustion in domestic and industrial premises and petrol and diesel engines. Although PM_{10} (particulate matter less than 10 µm) is the currently preferred measurement for particulate matter for which a standard is specified, the smaller particles ($PM_{2.5}$ and ultrafine particles) are becoming more important. These, together with benzene, butadiene and polycyclic aromatic hydrocarbons and heavy metals, are urban air pollutants. In the absence of significant wind, this can lead to temperature inversion effects in winter, causing local air pollution. Ozone is a secondary pollutant consequent on photochemical degradation. Photochemical 'smog' is a problem associated with cities, large numbers of vehicles, lack of air movement (wind) and high solar radiation. Photochemical 'smogs' can damage vegetation, including cash crops such as lettuce.

Acid rain or acid deposition is a regional problem dependent on the production of oxides of nitrogen and sulphur; sulphur oxides being formed from burning coal and oil in power stations, with the residence times of components in the atmosphere being in the order of several days. Lichens rapidly die out in areas where sulphur dioxide air pollution and acid rain occurs. However, often the effects of most concern are those affecting human health. Acid rain is also a major problem associated with the built environment.

Box 12.1 Ways in which pollutants adversely affect the atmosphere.

Tropospheric effects
- Degrading air quality (visibility, effects on human health and environmental effects), indoor and outdoor air, local and regional; includes 'smog' formation.
- Tropospheric ozone building.
- Acidification and eutrophication (acid rain, regional).

Stratospheric effects
- Stratospheric ozone layer depletion (polar 'ozone holes').
- Greenhouse warming potential (carbon dioxide).

Note
For further information, see Brimblecombe (1996) and Harrison (1990).

The greenhouse effect is a global problem associated with increasing levels of carbon dioxide in the troposphere. The burning of fossil fuels is one major factor implicated in the increase in atmospheric carbon dioxide. Other atmospheric components, such as methane and chlorofluorocarbons absorb outgoing radiation and therefore also contribute to the greenhouse effect. Organic chemicals may add to the greenhouse effect and tropospheric ozone levels. Ozone is formed in the troposphere from the oxidation of methane and carbon monoxide.

If a chemical contains fluorine and/or chlorine or bromine, then its ozone depletion potential will need to be quantified. These chemicals have very long (many years) residence times in the atmosphere and penetrate to the stratosphere. There, they cause the depletion of ozone from the polar regions of the stratospheric ozone layer in springtime. During the cold, dark polar winter, chemical reactions occur on the surface of atmospheric ice particles, leading to a build-up of chemicals that, on the coming of light, react with and deplete the ozone layer. This results in 'holes' in the ozone layer at the South Pole and considerable thinning at the North Pole. The ozone layer protects the earth from the harmful effects of ultraviolet radiation from the sun. Damage to vegetation is the environmental effect mediated by tropospheric pollutants.

Methods of assessment and management

Indoor and outdoor urban air pollution can be managed relatively locally. Exposure limits may constitute part of that management strategy.

Effects arising from longer range atmospheric pollution are going to be effects from relatively large releases of chemicals. Usually, the risks arising from the introduction of chemicals are first assessed judgementally. Existing risks often depend on calculations of the lifetimes in the relevant atmosphere, the inputs of the chemical and the atmospheric chemistry involved. These

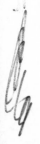

calculations therefore involve complicated models. In addition, as risk management often involves complicated international negotiations, there is a major international political process attached to the development of the assessment as well as to the management process. Control of the risks from greenhouse gases and stratospheric ozone-depleting chemicals depends on international agreement to reduce emissions, thus it requires agreement at the United Nations and implementation by regional groups, such as the EU, as well as by individual national governments.

Management of more local emissions can also be dealt with by control of emissions. National standards can be set for local and regional pollutants, and control exercised by seeking to reduce emission standards until the ambient medium standard can be met. Originally, the critical effect was seen as one on human health and environmental effects are only examined incidentally, so criteria for the acceptability of environmental standards were rarely required. Effects on vegetation are increasingly being considered, thus environmentally based criteria will be required when assessing and managing airborne risks.

References

Ballantyne, B., Marrs, T. and Syversen, T. (1999) *General and Applied Toxicology*, 2nd edn, London: Macmillan Reference.

Begon, M., Harpur, J.L. and Townsend, C.R. (1990) *Ecology: Individuals, Populations and Communities*, 2nd edn, Oxford: Blackwell.

Bell, S.G. and Codd, G.A. (1996) 'Detection, analysis and risk assessment of cyanobacterial toxins', in Hester, R.E. and Harrison, R.M. (eds) *Agricultural Chemicals in the Environment*, Issues in Environmental Science and Technology 5, Cambridge: Royal Society of Chemistry, pp. 109–22.

Bridges, J.W. (1990) 'Identification of toxic hazard', in Murray, V. (ed.) *Major Chemical Disasters – Medical Aspects of Management*, International Congress and Symposium series no. 155, London: Royal Society of Medicine.

Brimblecombe, P. (1996) *Air Composition and Chemistry*, Cambridge: Cambridge University Press.

Calabrese, E.J. (1983) *Principles of Animal Extrapolation*, New York: Wiley.

Calabrese, E.J., Beck, B.D. and Chappell, W.R. (1992) 'Does the animal-to-human uncertainty factor incorporate interspecies differences in surface area?', *Regulatory Toxicology and Pharmacology* 15, 172–9.

Calman, K.C. (1996) 'Cancer: science and society and the communication of risk', *British Medical Journal* 313, 799–802.

Calman, K.C. and Royston, G.H.D. (1997) 'Risk language and dialects', *British Medical Journal* 315, 939–42.

Chan, T.Y.K. (1997) 'Food delicacies as a cause of natural poisonings in Hong Kong', *Toxicology and Ecotoxicology News* 4, 124–6.

Chemical Incidents Response Service (2000) *The Chemical Incident Management Handbook: Practical Help for the Health and Emergency Services*. Medical Toxicology Unit, Guy's and St Thomas' Hospitals Trust. London: The Stationery Office.

Cohrssen, J.J. and Covello, V.T. (1989) *Risk Analysis: A Guide to the Principles and Methods for Analysing Health and Environmental Risks*, PB89-137772, Springfield, VA: National Technical Information Service.

Committee on Carcinogenicity (1991) *Guidelines for the Evaluation of Chemicals for Carcinogenicity*, Reps Health Social Subjects 42, London: HMSO.

Department of the Environment (1995) *A Guide to Risk Assessment and Risk Management for Environmental Protection*, London: HMSO.

Department of the Environment, Transport and the Regions (2000) *Guidance on the Interpretation of Major Accident for the Environment for the Proposed COMAH regulations*, London: The Stationary Office.

Dourson, M.L., Felter, S.P. and Robinson, D. (1996) 'Evolution of science based uncertainty factors in non-cancer risk assessment', *Regulatory Toxicology and Pharmacology* 24, 108–20.

Duffus, J.H. (1993) 'Glossary for chemists of terms used in toxicology', *Pure and Applied Chemistry* 65, 2003–122.

Duxbury, R. and Morton, S. (2000) *Blackstone's Strategy on Environmental Law*, 3rd edn, London: Blackstone Press.

ECETOC (1991) *Emergency Exposure Indices for Industrial Chemicals*, Technical report no. 43, Brussels: European Chemical Industry Ecology and Toxicology Centre.

ECETOC (1994) *Assessment of Non-occupational Exposure to Chemicals*, Technical report no. 58, Brussels: European Centre for Ecotoxicology and Toxicology.

ECETOC (1996) 'Risk assessment for carcinogens', monograph no. 24, Brussels: European Centre for Ecotoxicology and Toxicology of Chemicals.

ECETOC (1997) *Exposure Assessment in the Context of the EU Technical Guidance Documents on Risk Assessment of Substances*, ECETOC document no. 35, Brussels: European Centre for Ecotoxicology and Toxicology.

Fairhurst, S. (1995) 'The uncertainty factor in the setting of occupational exposure limits', *Annals of Occupational Hygiene* 39, 375–85.

Fairhurst, S. and Turner, R.M. (1993) 'Toxicological assessments in relation to major hazards', *Journal of Hazardous Materials* 33, 215–27.

Fawell, J. and Young, W. (1999) 'Exposure to chemicals through water', in Government/Research Councils Initiative on Risk Assessment and Toxicology (ed.) *Exposure Assessment in the Evaluation of Risks to Human Health*, Leicester: MRC Institute for Environment and Health.

Feron, V.J., van Bladeren, P.J. and Hermus, R.J.J. (1990) 'A viewpoint on the extrapolation of toxicological data from animals to man', *Food and Chemical Toxicology* 28, 783–8.

Franks, A.P., Harpur, P.J. and Bilo, M. (1996) 'The relationship between risk of death and risk of dangerous dose for toxic substances', *Journal of Hazardous Materials* 51, 11–14.

Gold, L.S., de Veciana, M., Backman, G.M. *et al.* (1986) 'Chronological supplement to the carcinogenic potency database: standardised results of animal bioassays published through December 1982', *Environmental Health Perspectives* 67, 161–200.

Gold, L.S., Manley, N.B., Slone, T.H. *et al.* (1992a) 'The fifth plot of the carcinogenic potency database: results of animal bioassays published in the literature through 1988 and the National Toxicology Program through 1989', *Environmental Health Perspectives* 100, 65–164.

Gold, L.S., Manley, N.B. and Ames, B.N. (1992b) 'Extrapolation of carcinogenicity between species', *Risk Analysis* 12, 579–88.

Gold, L.S., Sawyer, C.B., Magaw, R. *et al.* (1984) 'A carcinogenic potency database of the standardised results of animal bioassays', *Environmental Health Perspectives* 58, 9–319.

Gold, L.S., Slone, T.H., Backman, G.M. *et al*. (1987) 'Second chronological supplement to the carcinogenic potency database: standardised results of animal bioassays published through December 1984 and by the National Toxicology Program through May 1986', *Environmental Health Perspectives* 74, 237–329.

Gold, L.S., Slone, T.H., Backman, G.M. *et al*. (1990) 'Third chronological supplement to the carcinogenic potency database: standardised results of animal bioassays published through December 1986 and by the National Toxicology Program through June 1987', *Environmental Health Perspectives* 84, 215–86.

Government/Research Councils Initiative on Risk Assessment and Toxicology (1999a) *Risk Assessment Approaches Used by the UK Government for Evaluating Human Health Effects of Chemicals*, CR2, Leicester: MRC Institute for Environment and Health.

Government/Research Councils Initiative on Risk Assessment and Toxicology (1999b) *Risk Assessment Strategies in Relation to Population Sub-Groups*, CR3, Leicester: MRC Institute for Environment and Health.

Government/Research Councils Initiative on Risk Assessment and Toxicology (1999c) *Exposure Assessment in the Evaluation of Risk to Human Health*, CR5, Leicester: MRC Institute for Environment and Health.

Harrison, R.M. (1990) *Understanding our Environment*, 2nd edn, Cambridge: Royal Society of Chemistry.

Health and Safety Commission (1994) *Safety Data Sheets for Substances and Preparations Dangerous for Supply*, 2nd edn. Approved Code of Practice L62. Sudbury, UK: HSE Books.

Health and Safety Commission (1999) *Approved Guide to the Classification and Labelling of Substances and Preparations Dangerous for Supply*, 4th edn, Guidance on Regulations L100, Sudbury, UK: HSE Books.

Health and Safety Executive (1989) *The Tolerability of Risk from Nuclear Power Stations*, London: HMSO.

Health and Safety Executive (1992) *The Tolerability of Risk from Nuclear Power Stations*, 2nd edn, London: HMSO.

Health and Safety Executive (1994) *Risk Assessment of Notified New Substances*, technical guidance document, Sudbury, UK: HSE Books.

Health and Safety Executive (1999) *Reducing Risks, Protecting People*, discussion document, Sudbury, UK: HSE Books.

Hendy, J. and Ford, M. (1998) *Redgrave, Fife and Machin Health and Safety* (3rd edn with biennial updates), London: Butterworths.

HM Treasury (1996) 'The setting of safety standards. A report by an inter-departmental group and external advisors', available from the Public Enquiry Unit, HM Treasury, London.

Home Office (1994) *Dealing With Disasters*, 2nd edn, London: Her Majesty's Stationary Office.

HSE/MAFF (date not stated) *The Registration Handbook*, available from Pesticides Safety Directorate, Mallard House, Peasholme Green, York YO1 2PX. (Note: with the separation of the regulatory processes for plant protection products and biocides, this document is likely to become out of date shortly.)

Hughes, D. (1996) *Environmental Law*, 3rd edn, London: Butterworths.

IARC (1997) *IARC Monographs on the Evaluation of Carcinogenic Risk to Humans*, vol. 70, Lyon: International Agency for Research on Cancer.

ILGRA (1998) 'Risk communication: a guide to regulatory practice', available from ILGRA Secretariat, Health and Safety Executive, London.

Illing, H.P.A. (1989) 'Assessment of toxicology for major hazards: some concepts and problems', *Human and Experimental Toxicology* 10, 215–19.

Illing, H.P.A. (1991a) 'Extrapolating from toxicity data to occupational exposure limits: some considerations', *Annals of Occupational Hygiene* 35, 569–80.

Illing, H.P.A. (1991b) 'Possible risk considerations for toxic risk assessment', *Human and Experimental Toxicology* 10, 215–19.

Illing, H.P.A. (1993) 'Risk assessment and the evaluation of toxicity data: some ideas for discussion', *Arbete och Halsa* 15, 41–52.

Illing, H.P.A. (1999a) 'Are societal judgements being incorporated into the uncertainty factors used in toxicological risk assessment?', *Regulatory Toxicology and Pharmacology* 29, 300–8.

Illing, H.P.A. (1999b) 'Toxicology and disasters', in Ballantyne, B., Marrs, T.C. and Syversen, T. (eds) *General and Applied Toxicology*, 2nd edn, London: Macmillan Reference, pp. 1811–39.

IPCS (1978) *Principles and Methods for Evaluating the Toxicity of Chemicals.* Part 1. *Environmental Health Criteria 6*, Geneva: World Health Organisation.

IPCS (1987) *Principles for the Safety Assessment of Food Additives and Contaminants in Food. Environmental Health Criteria 70*, Geneva: World Health Organisation.

IPCS (1994) *Assessing Human Health Risks of Chemicals: Derivation of Guidance Values for Health-based Exposure Limits. Environmental Health Criteria 170*, Geneva: World Health Organisation.

IPCS (1999) *Public Health and Chemical Accidents. Guidance for National and Regional Policymakers in the Public/Environmental Roles*, WHO Collaborative Centre for an International Clearing House on Major Chemical Incidents, Cardiff: University of Wales Institute.

Jasanoff, S. (1992) 'Knowledge, responsibility and the safe use of chemicals', in Richardson, M.L. (ed.) *Risk Management of Chemicals*, London: Royal Society of Chemistry, pp. 337–67.

Johnson, E.M. (1988) 'Cross species extrapolations and the biologic basis for safety factor determinations in developmental toxicology', *Regulatory Toxicology and Pharmacology* 8, 22–36.

Jones, D. (1992) *Nomenclature for Hazard and Risk Assessment in the Process Industries*, 2nd edn, Rugby, UK: Institution of Chemical Engineers.

Kasperson, R.E., Renn, O., Slovic, P., Brown, H.S., Emel, J. *et al.* (1988) 'The social amplification of risk: a conceptual framework', *Risk Analysis* 8, 177–87.

Koundakjian, P. and Illing, H.P.A. (1992) 'Introduction', in Richardson, M.L. (ed.) *Risk Management for Chemicals*, Cambridge: Royal Society of Chemistry, pp 3–13.

Kramer, H.J., van den Ham, W.A., Slob, W. and Pieters, M.N. (1996) 'Conversion factors estimating indicative chronic no-observed-adverse-effect levels from short-term toxicity data', *Regulatory Toxicology and Pharmacology* 23, 249–55.

Langford, I., Marris, C., McDonald, A.L., Goldstein, H., Rasbah, J. and O'Riorden, T. (1999) 'Simultaneous analysis of individual and aggregate responses in psychometric data using multilevel modelling', *Risk Analysis* 19, 675–84.

Lehman, A.J. and Fitzhugh, O.G. (1954) '100 fold margin of safety', *Quarterly Bulletin of the Association of Food Drug Officials* 18, 33–5.

Lewalle, P. (1999) 'Risk assessment terminology – methodological considerations and provisional result: report of a WHO experiment', *Terminology Standardisation and Harmonisation* 11 (1–4), 1–28.

Lovell, D.P. and Thomas, G. (1996) 'Quantitative risk assessment and the limitations of the linearized multistage model', *Human and Experimental Toxicology* 15, 87–104.

McDonald, A.L., Fielder, R.J., Diggle, G.E., Tennant, D.R. and Fisher, C.E. (1996) 'Carcinogens in food: priorities for regulation', *Human and Experimental Toxicology* 15, 739–46.

Mackay, D., Paterson, S. and Shiu, W.Y. (1992) 'Generic models for evaluating the regional fate of chemicals', *Chemosphere* 24, 695–717.

Mackay D., Di Guardo, A., Paterson, S. and Cowan, C.E. (1996a) 'Evaluating the environmental fate of a variety of types of chemicals using the EQC model', *Environmental Toxicology and Chemistry* 15, 1627–37.

Mackay, D., Di Guardo, A., Paterson, S., Kiksi, G. and Cowan, C.E. (1996b) 'Assessing the fate of new and existing chemicals: a five stage process', *Environmental Toxicology and Chemistry* 15, 1618–26.

Marris, C., Langford, I., Saunderson, T. and O'Riorden, T. (1997) 'Exploring the "Psychometric Paradigm": comparisons between aggregate and individual analyses', *Risk Analysis* 17, 303–12.

Maynard, R.L., Cameron, K.M., Fielder, R., McDonald, A. and Wadge, A. (1995) 'Setting air quality standards for carcinogens: an alternative to mathematical quantitative risk assessment – Discussion paper', *Human and Experimental Toxicology* 14, 175–86.

MHAP (1993) 'Phosgene toxicity', major hazards monograph, Rugby: Institution of Chemical Engineers.

Murray, V. (ed.) (1990) *Major Chemical Disasters – Medical Aspects of Management*, International Congress and Symposium series no. 155, London: Royal Society of Medicine.

National Research Council (1983) *Risk Assessment in the Federal Government: Managing the Process*, Washington, DC: National Academy Press.

National Research Council (1994) *Science and Judgement in Risk Assessment*. Washington, DC: National Academy Press.

National Research Council (1996) *Understanding Risk*. Washington, DC: National Academy Press.

Niemeyer, R. (1993) 'Management of OELs in the United States', *Arbete och Halsa* 15, 33–40.

OECD (1981) *Guidelines to the Toxicity Testing of Chemicals* (updated periodically), Paris: Organisation for Economic Co-operation and Development.

Otway, H.J. and von Winterfeldt, D. (1982) 'Beyond acceptability of risk: on the social acceptability of technologies', *Policy Sciences* 14, 247–56.

Pepelco, W.E. (1987) 'Feasibility of route extrapolation in risk assessment', *British Journal of Industrial Medicine* 44, 649–51.

Pepelko, W.E. and Withey, J.R. (1985) 'Methods for route-to-route extrapolation of dose', *Toxicology and Industrial Health* 1, 153–70.

Pesticides Safety Directorate (1986) 'UK predictive operator exposure model (POEM). Estimation of exposure and absorption by spray operators', available from Pesticides Safety Directorate, York.

Pesticides Safety Directorate (1992) 'UK predictive operator exposure model (POEM). A users guide', available from Pesticides Safety Directorate, York.

Peto, R., Pike, M.C., Pike, L., Bernstein, L., Gold, L.S. and Ames, B.N. (1984) 'The TD50: a proposed general convention for the numerical description of the carcinogenic potential of chemicals in chronic exposure animal studies', *Environmental Health Perspectives* 58, 1–8.

Presidential/Congressional Commission on Risk Assessment and Risk Management (1997) *Framework for Environmental Health Risk Management. Final Report*, Washington, DC: Presidential/Congressional Commission on Risk Assessment and Risk Management.

Rees, N. (1999) 'Dietary exposure assessment', in Government/Research Councils Initiative on Risk Assessment and Toxicology (ed.) *Exposure Assessment in the Evaluation of Risks to Human Health*, Leicester: MRC Institute for Environment and Health.

Renn, O. (1998) 'Three decades of risk research: accomplishments and new challenges', *Journal of Risk Research*, 1, 49–71.

Renwick, A.G. (1993) 'Data derived safety factors for the evaluation of food additives and environmental chemicals', *Food Additives and Contaminants* 10, 275–306.

Renwick, A.G. (1995) 'The use of an additional safety or uncertainty factor for nature of toxicity in the estimation of acceptable daily intake and tolerable daily intake values', *Regulatory Toxicology and Pharmacology* 22, 250–61.

Renwick, A.G. (1998) 'Toxicokinetics in infants and children in relation to ADI and TDI', *Food Additives and Contaminants* 15 (Suppl.), 17–35.

Renwick, A.G. and Lazarus, N. (1998) 'Human variability and noncancer risk assessment – an analysis of the default uncertainty factor', *Regulatory Toxicology and Pharmacology* 27, 3–20.

Royal Commission on Environmental Pollution (1998) *Setting Environmental Standards. Twenty-first Report*, London: The Stationary Office.

Royal Society Study Group (1983) *Risk Assessment*, London: Royal Society.

Royal Society Study Group (1992) *Risk: Analysis, Perception and Management*, London: Royal Society.

Rubery, E.D., Barlow, S.M. and Stedman, J.H. (1990) 'Criteria for setting quantitative estimates of chemicals in food in the UK', *Food Additives and Contaminants* 7, 287–302.

Sharratt, M. (1988) 'Assessing risks from data on other exposure routes', *Regulatory Toxicology and Pharmacology* 8, 399–407.

Shaw, I.C. and Chadwick, J. (1998) *Principals of Environmental Toxicology*, London: Taylor and Francis.

Slovic, P. (1997) 'Trust, emotion, sex, politics and science: surveying the risk assessment battlefield', in Bazerman, M., Messik, D., Tenbrunsel, A. and Wade-Benzoni, K. (eds) *Environment, Ethics and Behaviour*, San Francisco: The New Lexington Press (reprinted in *Risk Analysis* 19, 689–702, 1999).

Try, P.M. and Price, G.J. (1995) 'Sewage and industrial effluents', in *Waste Treatment and Disposal*, Issues in Environmental Science and Technology 3, Cambridge: Royal Society of Chemistry, pp. 17–41.

Voisin, E.M., Ruthsatz, M., Collins, J.M. and Hoyle, P.C. (1990) 'Extrapolation of animal toxicity to humans', *Regulatory Toxicology and Pharmacology* 12, 107–16.

Wells, G. (1997) *Major Hazards and Their Management*, Rugby: Institution of Chemical Engineers.

WHO/FAO (1995) *Application of Risk Analysis to Food Standards Issues*, report of a joint World Health Organisation/Food and Agriculture Organisation (WHO/FAO) expert consultation, WHO/FNU/FOS/95.3, Geneva: WHO.

Wilson, H.K. (1999) 'Biological monitoring values for occupational exposure: a United Kingdom perspective', *Archives of Occupational and Environmental Health* 72, 274–8.

Withey, J.R. (1987) 'Approaches to route extrapolation', in Tardiff, R.G. and Rodricks, J.V. (eds) *Toxic Substances and Human Risk*, New York: Plenum Press.

Woodward, K.N. and Dayan, A.D. (1990) 'Strength of meaning – strong words and a certain message?', *Human and Experimental Toxicology* 9, 53–4.

Appendix 1   Hazard assessment for labelling: the European Union system

Within the European economic area, there is a uniform system for classification of the hazards of industrial chemicals for use with labels and safety data sheets. Similar requirements also exist in other parts of the world, notably the USA. The system is hazard based – the risk assessment is a follow through when the information provided in the materials safety data sheets is examined in the light of the particular exposure circumstances pertaining to the workstation or discharge route. The aim is to ensure that information is passed down the supply chain from manufacturer to user (industrial, professional or amateur/domestic) and through to final disposal as waste. The areas covered include physicochemical information, information on mammalian toxicity and information on environmental effects. Associated with the 'risk (R) phrases' (which describe hazard in order to suggest the potential risks that might be posed) are 'safety (S) phrases' suggesting basic precautions to be considered when using or disposing of the chemical. Some R phrases contain an element of dose–response. These include those associated with human health acute toxicity and irritancy and corrosivity for skin and eye, as well as toxicity to aquatic organisms. Others are simple yes/no triggers to labelling, as with skin sensitisation and respiratory irritancy and sensitisation on the human health phrases, and the phrases associated with non-aquatic toxicity on the environmental side. Carcinogenicity, mutagenicity and reproductive toxicity is 'quality of evidence' based. The category to which a chemical is assigned depends on the nature of the evidence, not on potency. The full list of R phrases is in Box A1.1.

This type of scheme may be extended to 'preparations' (mixtures of chemicals, in reality the more realistic situation as far as marketing is concerned). Although experimental studies can be used to examine the properties of these preparations, these would need to be very extensive if every potential preparation were to be fully tested for toxicity and ecotoxicity. Thus, there are usually administrative procedures for choosing the R phrases based on the amounts of classified chemicals present.

Box A1.1 Risk phrases for classification and labelling.

Physicochemical properties

R1   Explosive when dry
R2   Risk of explosion by shock, friction, fire or other sources of ignition
R3   Extreme risk of explosion by shock, friction, fire or other sources of ignition
R4   Forms very sensitive explosive metallic compounds
R5   Heating may cause an explosion
R6   Explosive with or without contact with air
R7   May cause fire
R8   Contact with combustible material may cause fire
R9   Explosive when mixed with combustible material
R10   Flammable
R11   Highly flammable
R12   Extremely flammable
R14   Reacts violently with water
R15   Contact with water liberates extremely flammable gases
R16   Explosive when mixed with oxidising substances
R17   Spontaneously flammable in air
R18   In use may form flammable/explosive vapour-air mixtures
R19   May form explosive peroxides
R30   Can become highly flammable in use
R44   Risk of explosion if heated under confinement

Mammalian toxicity (classification on the basis of health effects)

Acute toxicity
R20   Harmful by inhalation
R21   Harmful in contact with skin
R22   Harmful if swallowed
R23   Toxic by inhalation
R24   Toxic in contact with skin
R25   Toxic if swallowed
R26   Very toxic by inhalation
R27   Very toxic in contact with skin
R28   Very toxic if swallowed
R39   Danger of very serious irreversible effects after a single exposure
R40   Possible risk of irreversible effects

Irritancy and corrosivity
R34   Causes burns
R35   Causes severe burns
R36   Irritating to eyes
R37   Irritating to respiratory system
R38   Irritating to skin
R41   Risk of serious damage to eyes

Sensitisation
R42   May cause sensitisation by inhalation
R43   May cause sensitisation by skin contact

Carcinogenicity, mutagenicity and reproductive toxicity
R40   Possible risk of irreversible effects
R45   May cause cancer
R46   May cause heritable genetic damage
R49   May cause cancer by inhalation
R60   May impair fertility
R61   May cause harm to the unborn child
R62   Possible risk of impaired fertility
R63   Possible risk of harm to the unborn child

Additional risk phrases
R29   Contact with water liberates toxic gas
R31   Contact with acid liberates toxic gas
R32   Contact with water liberates very toxic gas
R33   Danger of cumulative effects
R64   May cause harm to breast-fed babies
R66   Repeated exposure may cause skin dryness or cracking
R67   Vapours may cause drowsiness and dizziness

Environmental effects

Aquatic environment
R50   Very toxic to aquatic organisms
R51   Toxic to aquatic organisms
R52   Harmful to aquatic organisms
R53   May cause long-term adverse effects in the aquatic environment

Non-aquatic environment
R54   Toxic to flora
R55   Toxic to fauna
R56   Toxic to soil organisms
R57   Toxic to bees
R58   May cause long-term adverse effects in the environment

Effects in the stratosphere
R59   Dangerous for the ozone layer

From the Health and Safety Commission (1999).

Index

abiotic removal processes 124–5
acceptability of risk 36, 42
accidental risk 14, 15
acid rain 135
administrative law 29
adverse effect level, non-observable
    75–6
agencies (US system of) 26–7
Agenda 21 19
Agriculture, Fisheries and Food, UK
    Ministry of 28
air quality standard/objective 39
ALARP (risk as low as reasonably
    practicable) 38
analysis of toxicological risk, process
    of 61
animal testing 65–6
anticipatable risks 14, 15
aquatic (and non-aquatic) environment
    147
articulation of values 55–6
assessment of risk
    atmosphere, effects on 136–7;
        hazards, major 105, 108–10;
        philosophical framework 32, 34;
        of risk 8–10; two camps on, vii;
        UK bodies for 28–9; see also
        evaluation of risk; exposure
        assessment; perception of risk;
        toxicological assessment
    acid rain 135; assessment of risk
        136–7; atmospheric cycling
        processes 135; atmospheric
        structure 133–4; chemicals as
        pollutants 134–6; greenhouse
        effect, 136; management of risk
        136–7; ozone depletion 136;
        photochemical smog, 135;

stratospheric effects 136;
    tropospheric effects 136; urban air
    135; see also environment, effects
    of
attitudes to risk, differences in 45–7

BAT (best available technique) 38
BBDR (biologically based dose–
    response) 91
benchmark dose (BMD) 74, 75, 76
bioaccumulation/concentration/
    magnification 127–8
biological organisation/toxicants 2–3
BPEO (best practicable environmental
    option) 38
British Toxicology Society, vii
broadly acceptable risk
    explicit decisions on 55–6;
        perception of risk 45, 47–8, 49,
        55–6; toxicity, human health
        evaluation 85, 86
    bureaucrats and risk 48

carcinogenicity 84–90, 147
carcinogens, classification of 87
cellular toxicology 3
channel problems, communication of
    risk 49
chemicals
    airborne 109; atmospheric pollutants
        134–6; bioconcentration of 119;
        environmental pollutants 124; in
        food 98–100; human exposure
        after major accident 108; OECD
        test guidelines for 66, 68–9;
        physicochemical properties, 146;
        risks of exposure to 15, 18;
        toxicants 2; see also hazards

Henry's law, biodegradation and 124, 125
hierarchy of risk 47
Home Office (UK) 29

ILGRA (Interdepartmental Liaison Group on Risk Assessment) 51, 54
indicator species, toxicity in 126–7, 130–1
individual concern 46
individual risk 5, 8, 59, 60
individualism 47, 48
information sources 65, 70; see also data
inhalation studies 73
Institution of Chemical Engineers 7
interactions, biological systems and substances 3
Interagency Organisation for the Management of Chemicals 3
interindividual variations 79
International Agency for Research on Cancer (IARC) 86, 87
international bodies 15–19
International Committee on Harmonisation (ICH) 66
international law 21–4
International Maritime Organisation 24
international regulation 27
interspecies variations 78
IPPC/IPPM 19, 38
irritancy 146
IUAPC Commission on Toxicology 6

land-use planning criteria 112–13
legal context
  administrative law 29; civil law 29; development of legislation 21, 22–3; European law 21–4; international law 21–4; statute law 20–5; UK law 20–1; UK legislative instruments 23; US law 24–5; see also organisational context
lethality, boundary conditions for 116
licensing process 62–3
life-cycle analysis 41
LOAEL (lowest observed adverse effect level) 74–6, 79, 83
  local government 19; see also government

Major Hazards Assessment Panel 116
mammalian toxicity 146
management of risk
  accidental risk 14, 15; anticipatable risks 14, 15; atmosphere, effects on 136–7; chemicals, risks of exposure to 15, 18; communication and 15, 54–5; companies and 19; definitions of 13–14; description of 8–10; environmental risks 14, 17; health risks 13–14; international bodies 15–19; local government and 19; national bodies 15–19; objective risk 14, 16; occupational health risks, 14; pathways, emission to take up 18; perceived risk 14, 16; philosophical framework 35; pollution and 14, 17; preventative approach to 18–19; product/process safety 17, 18–19; public health risks 14, 16; standards 17–18, 30, 38; statistical risk 14, 16; toxicological assessment 62–3
management systems 25–9
'margin of exposure' approach 83
maximum exposure limit 39
measurements of exposure 96–7, 102
media, meeting the needs of the 52–3
message problems in communication of risk 49
modifying factors 76, 78
molecular toxicology 3
monitoring environmental exposure 131
mutagenicity 84, 147

National Academy of Sciences 59–61
national bodies 15–19
National Research Council (US) 25, 32
NOAEL (no observable adverse effect level) 74–7, 79–85, 96, 100, 103
non-stochastic effects 73–4
Notification of New Substances Regulations (1993) 23

objective risk
  management of risk 14, 16; perception of risk 43–4, 56
occupational exposure
  health risks 14; levels 82; standard 39
OECD/IPCS harmonisation project 6,